The Skinny Book
Second Edition

Includes the
6-Step Weight Loss Diet™

The "80% knowledge
& 20% effort"
diet and lifestyle

Ayaz Virji, MD

Verona Publishing, Inc.
P.O. Box 24071
Edina, Minnesota 55424

www.veronapublishing.com

Verona Publishing is pleased to present
The Skinny Book Second Edition.

If you are interested in purchasing more copies or if you are interested in books on other topics, contact Verona Publishing.
Books may be ordered online at www.veronapublishing.com.

When ordering in bulk, e-mail us the type and number of books required at info@veronapublishing.com.

If you have questions or comments, contact us at info@veronapublishing.com.

Design and layout by Kathy Harestad, www.KathyArt.com

The Skinny Book Second Edition – first published 2008

©2008 by Ayaz Virji, MD

Published by Verona Publishing, Inc., P.O. Box 24071, Edina, Minnesota 55424

Library of Congress Cataloging-in-Publication Data:

Library of Congress Control Number: 2007928681

ISBN : 978-0-976-90312-3

Verona Publishing, Inc.
P.O. Box 24071
Edina, Minnesota 55424

www.veronapublishing.com

The ideas and methods expressed in this work represent the opinions of the author only. Before starting any weight loss program you should first consult with your doctor. This publication was made to be informative on the topic of weight management, but in no way represents a replacement for individualized medical care from your doctor. Neither the publisher nor the author claim any responsibility for liability or harm incurred on the reader secondary to utilization of any of the advice or recommendations of any part of this book.

Certain medical concepts and mechanisms of action of human physiology have been simplified in order to promote understanding for the greatest number of people. By doing this, it is the author's intention not to let medical jargon or complexity interfere with the major points conveyed in this text. It should be understood that the advancement of medical science is based on the development and applications of theoretical principles. These principles are constantly undergoing re-analysis and may change over time as scientific understanding of the particular principle or topic develops and matures.

Preface to Second Edition

Like every other field of medicine, bariatric (weight loss) medicine is constantly being updated with exciting new research and scientific publications. As we learn more about the many different factors affecting our population's current unhealthy weight epidemic, we also learn more about how to avoid it. That was my inspiration for writing this second edition of The Skinny Book.

There are over 6,000 scientific studies published a year on the topics of nutrition and weight loss. We are uncovering the various ways that macronutrients (protein, fat, carbohydrates, and alcohol) and micronutrients (vitamins, minerals, and phytonutrients) actually affect our body's fat burning hormones. In addition, we are learning more and more about the importance of serving size on calorie intake, the importance of non-exercise activity thermogenesis (NEAT) on daily calorie burn, the role of certain stomach hormones on appetite regulation and how to control them.....The list goes on and on!

Since publishing the first edition, probably the most common comment I received from my readers was that they wanted to see the actual 6-Step Weight Loss Diet and and to understand how it is used on our clinic population. The goal for the first edition was to inspire the reader to learn more about unhealthy weight and how it affects overall health in general. Weight loss can no longer be accepted as something an individual does to strictly improve his or her looks or self-image. It must also be regarded as something an individual does to prevent significant medical conditions including heart disease, diabetes, and cancer. In the first edition, I tried to convey this idea the best I could in an easy-to-read format as well as provide various alternative diets that currently exist on the market and my opinions about them.

In this edition, you will find the 6-Step Weight Loss diet explained in detail and will learn how it works to enhance your fat burning hormones and reduce your fat storing hormones. We continue to have tremendous success with it in our clinic population and feel that you can too. I describe our unique multi-dimensional nutritional analysis technique and how we use it to categorize food to make weight loss as easy as possible. Our diet has been described as "80% knowledge and 20% effort." Just read the book in its entirety and you will find out why. We have added a few extra sections including: discussion on the various hormones involved in weight loss and how to control them; common medications that cause weight gain; popular over-the-counter diet aids; and 6-Step Weight Loss original recipes. I hope you enjoy reading this second edition as much as I have enjoyed writing it.

Ayaz Virji, MD

Table of Contents

Unhealthy Weight as an Epidemic

When we speak of medical diseases the first thing that comes to our mind is heart disease, stroke, and cancer. And why not? These diseases are the leading causes of death and suffering nationwide, and perhaps worldwide. We all have friends or family members who are suffering from or were lost to a heart attack or a various type of cancer. We almost never hear of those people who are suffering from or who died of being overweight. That would be absurd, right?

Wrong! Unhealthy weight is one of the leading causes of death and suffering in this country (1,2). Unhealthy weight is a major risk factor for heart disease, stroke, diabetes, colon cancer, breast cancer, ulcer diseases, gallbladder disease, osteoarthritis, major depressive disorders, and chronic pain disorders to name a few. Overweight patients suffer from more chronic medical conditions than patients of normal weight and body mass index. Sadly, it is harder to perform major surgeries on such patients because of anatomical barriers.

Given the above information and the fact that over 60% of American adults suffer from unhealthy weight, I think I've shown you that obesity is an epidemic in this country that can lead to significant medical complications and even death (3). It acts as a thread that binds together an assortment of diseases. Therefore, weight management issues are no longer of crucial importance only to the medical community but to the nation as a whole.

I hope I have convinced you, the reader, that unhealthy weight as a disease is at the same level of importance as heart disease, diabetes, and even breast cancer. In fact, it happens to be an independent risk factor for all three of these. Dealing with weight management is like repairing a shipping vessel before sending it out to sea. Treating a heart attack or stroke is like rescuing the passengers from the sinking ship. Why not work on measures to prevent the catastrophe rather than on the effects of the catastrophe? This is a simple analogy. Nevertheless, the point remains that by "repairing" unhealthy weight, the prevalence of heart disease, strokes, diabetes, and cancer are guaranteed to significantly decline in this country.

As a physician, I deal with obesity and weight management on a daily basis. My methods have been extremely successful in helping a large proportion of my patients "repair" their unhealthy weight. Unfortunately, in the medical field, weight management does not get attributed the amount of attention and time it really deserves.

For example, in primary care we deal with upper respiratory infections, heart disease, diabetes, fractures, rashes, newborn exams, liver disease, asthma, migraine headaches, etc. In a typical day, your average family physician will deal with all of the above plus about 20-30 more medical issues for patients. On top of that is the endless amount of paperwork, charting, and coding required by insurance companies and the legal system that has to be dealt with. It can be quite overwhelming.

You can imagine your average physician's response when a patient inquires about weight loss. "Diet and exercise" is the answer. But what exactly does that mean? What diet is best for you? How will you get there? What medications may be contributing to your weight? How will weight be maintained? What type of medical surveillance or technology can help?

These are all issues that need to be thoroughly addressed before weight loss can be achieved and maintained successfully. Your physician will be so busy dealing with many different, more immediate problems, as well as fulfilling mandatory administrative paperwork, that he may show little enthusiasm for questions about your weight if you do it as an after-thought.

Weight management requires a significant amount of time and

energy from both sides, patient and doctor. As a patient, you would not end a visit with your doctor by saying, "Oh, and about my chest pain." Weight concerns, like chest pain, merit the complete attention of your doctor and should be the sole focus of your visit when addressing it.

The Purpose
of This Book

The purpose of this book is to introduce you to my 6-Step Weight Loss program. This book will help give you the critical information you need to help you lose weight in a healthy and sustainable way. The 6-Step Weight Loss Diet, which is reviewed later, has been described as "80% knowledge and 20% effort." This is due to its simplicity and relative ease of use. In order to be successful you must read this book from cover to cover and understand what is being taught.

I will take you through the physiology of weight reduction and weight loss maintenance. You will learn about the many medical conditions associated with unhealthy weight and more importantly how they may have slowed down your weight loss success in the past. We will use principles of biochemistry as well as psychology to help you achieve your goal. Patients in my clinic have a very high success rate for weight loss and long term weight loss maintenance. I will do my best to help teach you all you need to know to experience the same level of success.

The best part about this book is that you're going to learn all you need to know in record time! I have purposely made this book as compact as possible for quick reading and easy referencing. You don't need a 500 page book to describe to you how to lose weight. In the words of Albert Einstein, "Things should be made as simple as possible, but not simpler."

Now, let us begin our journey.

Why My Methods Work: The Multi-factorial Approach

I n the Medical field, the majority of diseases we treat have multi-factorial etiologies. What this means is that there is no one thing causing them. Instead, many different things are involved to cause you to develop a certain disease. Consider the following examples.

Heart disease is not caused by increased cholesterol alone. Other modifiable risk factors besides high cholesterol that lead to heart disease include: OBESITY, high blood pressure, sedentary lifestyle, diabetes, and elevated homocysteine levels (family history, age, and gender are not modifiable risk factors). Factors that lead to colon cancer include: OBESITY, high-fat, low-fiber diet, chronic constipation, and family history. Factors involved in gallstone formation include: OBESITY, age, fertility status, and gender. The list goes on and on. We could fill an entire book just listing all the specific risk factors for the different diseases out there. The point being, no one particular thing has total say over whether or not you develop or can control a certain disease. There are many forces at work, and successful disease control involves recognition and treatment of the many different variables involved.

Being overweight is no different. Risk factors include: a sedentary lifestyle, poor diet, certain medical conditions (hypothyroidism, anemia, insomnia,..), certain medications, and depression. I would also extend this list to include unhealthy cognitive barriers and detrimental behavior patterns. The 6-Step Weight Loss Program deals with every modifiable aspect of unhealthy weight not just diet and exercise alone, which is why it is so successful. Here is a summary of how it is done:

Step 1: Medical Screening: The first step is to ensure that you are healthy enough to begin an active weight loss program and to ensure that there is no underlying medical condition involved that may have sabotaged your weight loss efforts in the past. In addition, we'll review some common medications which can slow down weight loss. You will need your doctor's help with this.

Step 2: Patient Education: Knowledge is power. Once you see how the pieces of the puzzle fit, your goal of weight management becomes much easier to obtain. We do this by teaching you about certain key hormones involved in weight loss and what you can do to control them.

Step 3: 6-Step Weight Loss Diet: Dieting does not have to be painful. Our diet has been described as "80% knowledge and 20% effort." We have a unique *multi-dimensional nutritional analysis* technique we use to make the diet as simple and painless as possible. This will likely not only be the most effective diet you have ever tried, but also one of the easiest!

Step 4: Cognitive Principles: Certain misconceptions about weight loss create significant barriers to weight management. We will eradicate these and prevent them from returning.

Step 5: Behavioral Issues: We'll discuss some key, high yield behavioral patterns specific to healthy weight management including: understanding eating cues, effective activity modification, and social support.

Step 6: Weight Loss Maintenance: Losing weight is half the battle. Maintaining the lost weight is the other half (and arguably the more important). We'll review the 6-Step Weight Maintenance Diet in this section as well as key weight loss maintenance strategies.

Now, let's begin the 6-Step Weight Loss Program. Success is awaiting you at the turn of a page!

Step 1:
Medical Screening

I have already shown you that obesity is related to many diseases and by preventing it you will add many quality years to your life. Before you begin the process of weight management, you need to be certain that you don't have any medical conditions that are going to slow down your weight loss. Going to your physician and getting a Complete Physical Exam (your doctor may refer to this as a CPE) is the first step. This should include a head-to-toe exam, appropriate preventive screening, and lab work. The lab work will include a complete blood count (CBC), a complete metabolic profile (CMP), a fasting lipid profile (which is the technical term for a complete cholesterol panel), and thyroid level (TSH) (Table 1). Tell your physician that you are beginning a new weight management program and you want to be sure you are healthy enough to do so. Annual physical exams are very informative to both patients and physicians, and I would recommend them to everyone, whether you are trying to lose weight or not.

Table 1: Important lab tests prior to _ANY_ weight loss program

Complete Blood Count (CBC)
> Will check for anemia or vitamin deficiency.
> Helps guide more advanced nutritional supplementation if needed.

Complete Metabolic Profile (CMP)
> Will ensure healthy kidney and liver function and screen for abnormal blood sugars commonly associated with being overweight.

Fasting Lipid Profile (FLP)
> Baseline complete cholesterol test, looks at both good and bad cholesterol. Cholesterol is bound to improve with your weight loss; so it's helpful to get your starting point.

Thyroid Test (TSH)
> Will screen normal thyroid function. Poor thyroid function may slow down weight loss.

A complete blood count (CBC) helps screen for anemia and vitamin deficiencies. It does so by looking at the size, shape, and color of the red blood cells, which can vary with certain blood disorders and nutritional deficiencies.

Unhealthy weight is the most common cause of a certain liver disease called NASH (non-alcoholic steatohepatitis). This is where fatty acids accumulate in liver cells leading to inflammation and scarring. This can be a risk factor for significant liver disease later in life. The complete metabolic profile (CMP) will screen for NASH. NASH generally improves with weight loss. If you have NASH, once you lose the weight your doctor can reorder the test for you and you will see the improvement for yourself. The CMP will also screen for elevated blood sugar and certain kidney diseases.

Knowing your kidney function is important and gives us a baseline measure of the various minerals and salts in your blood as well. Certain diets will make the kidneys work a little harder for a short period of time so you want to ensure they are ready to handle the task. In most otherwise healthy people this is not a problem. In people with compromised kidney function this needs to be watched closely.

Checking your cholesterol is very important as well. According to the National Cholesterol Education Program (NCEP) guidelines all people above the age of twenty should be screened for high cholesterol. If you are overweight it is likely that your cholesterol is also high. You need to know your cholesterol levels. Specifically, you need to know what your levels are for LDL (bad cholesterol) and HDL (good cholesterol). For your LDL, the lower the better; For your HDL, the higher the better. No matter where your cholesterol is now, it's almost guaranteed to improve once the weight comes off. If you are on a cholesterol lowering medication, you may even be able to reduce the dose or discontinue it completely once you've lost the weight. Your doctor can explain to you what your specific cholesterol goals are since it varies from person to person.

Hypothyroidism (or low thyroid hormone level) will slow down your body's metabolism. Symptoms include obesity, constipation, fatigue, dry skin, and hair loss. Your doctor will order a TSH level (thyroid stimulating hormone), which gives a reasonable measure of your thyroid gland's function.

If you have clinical depression or another mood disorder, you need to discuss that with your doctor and get treatment first. Depressive disorders can cause what we call psychomotor retardation which basically makes you and your body move with a general slowing and lack of energy. This will slow your metabolism and your weight loss, not to mention be bad for your overall health in general. There are some great medical treatments out there for depression that will make you feel better and also add years to your life. An important medical study called the SADHEART Trial showed that in patients who suffered a heart attack and who had their depression treated lived much longer and were less likely to suffer another heart attack than those who had untreated depression.

Actually, effectively managing your weight with the 6-Step Weight Loss Program will have a positive effect on your mood and energy level overall (4). You'll find that as you lose weight your depression will get better as well. Nevertheless, we do not want any psychological issues hindering our weight management program.

Traditional approaches to weight loss do not even consider these very important medical and psychological factors. All patients in my weight management clinic get a complete physical exam (CPE), appropriate lab work, and general medical screening to prepare them for the upcoming weight loss and maintenance. This is one of the reasons the program is so successful. You need to know how your weight is affecting your own health. We need to be sure there is nothing predisposing you to failure on a biological or psychological level.

One patient who came to see me for some help in weight loss who said he had tried everything and had known nothing but failure his entire life. I enrolled him in my program. I checked his thyroid level which happened to be low, and I corrected it. We went through the program together, and he successfully lost over 30 lbs. He is down to his ideal body weight and has kept it off. He is currently in step 6 (Weight Maintenance) which is lifelong and prevents weight rebound.

I had another overweight patient come to me insisting that her thyroid be checked. She claimed she was doing everything right but not losing the weight. She had already had her thyroid checked earlier in the year, and it was normal. When I reviewed this with her she began to cry. I immediately noted her cognitive barrier to weight loss. I gave her cognitive and behavioral therapy, enrolled her in my program, and she lost 50 lbs and has thus far kept it off.

Now, the last piece of the puzzle that needs to be sorted out during the medical visit: Medications that may be stalling your weight loss success. I'm going to preface this part of the talk by saying that that you should NEVER stop, change, or alter in any way your current medication regimen without the supervision of your doctor. You will definitely need your doctor's help and input on this in order to modify your medication regimen to be most favorable to help you achieve long term weight loss success. I must also emphasize that there are times when it may not be possible to change your medication.

For example, if you are someone who has had a heart attack, then you may be on a particular blood pressure medication that may slow down weight loss. There is nothing we can do about that because that medication may be preventing you from having another heart attack. In such cases, we just work around it.

In the medical field, instead of talking about specific medications, we discuss them as a part of a "class of medication." This helps to simplify things and avoid long lists of medications that are hard to remember anyway. Refer to Table 2 for a review of some common medical conditions along with the "class of medication" used to treat those conditions. If you are on medication for any of the discussed medical conditions and are not sure if it is in any of the specific classes mentioned, then just ask your doctor or pharmacist and they will clarify that for you. I refer to the medications as either weight positive (slows down weight loss); weight neutral (has no effect on weight); or weight negative (helps with weight loss). Remember, any changes in medications that you take will have to involve your medical provider and should not be instituted just by reading this book.

Table 2: Common medications and their effect on weight.

Clinical Condition	Weight Positive Medications	Weight Neutral Medications	Weight Negative Medications
Diabetes	glimepiride (*Amaryl*®) glyburide (*Micronase*®, *DiaBeta*®) pioglitazone (*Actos*®) rosiglitazone (*Avandia*®) repaglinide (*Prandin*®) insulin (*Novolin*®, *Humulin*®, *Lantus*®)	sitagliptin (*Januvia*™)	metformin (*Gucophage*®) exenatide (*Byatta*®) pramlintide (*Symlin*®) acarbose (*Precose*®)
Blood Pressure	atenolol (*Tenormin*®) Metoprolol (*Lopressor*®, *Toprol XL*®) propranolol (*Inderal*®)	carvedilol (*Coreg*®) labetalol (*Trandate*®) diltiazem (*Cardizem*®) verapamil (*Calan*®, *Veralan PM*®)	hydrochlorothiazide (*HCTZ*) chlorthalidone (*Hygroton*®) lisinopril (*Zestril*®) benazepril (*Lotensin*®) enalapril (*Vasotec*®) quinapril (*Accupril*®) preindopril (*Aceon*®)
Migraines	atenolol (*Tenormin*®) metoprolol (*Lopressor*®, *Toprol XL*®) propranolol (*Inderal*®)	diltiazem (*Cardizem*®) verapamil (*Calan*®, *Veralan PM*®)	topiramate (*Topamax*®)
Depression	paroxetine (*Paxil*®) fluoxetine (*Prozac*®) citalopram (*Celexa*®)	sertraline (*Zoloft*®) venlefaxine (*Effexor*®)	buproprion (*Wellbutrin XL*®)

All right, that about does it for the very brief review of common medications that may affect your weight. Remember, if you are not sure if you are taking any of the specific classes of medications mentioned then just ask your doctor or pharmacist. Medical screening and surveillance are important parts of the weight management package. Now that you understand their significance, you see why many weight loss programs fail in helping you lose the weight or keep the weight off. You need your doctor's help in identifying these barriers so you can cross them and move on. Now, let's move on to Step 2.

Step 2:
Patient Education

All right, hold on to your hats! Knowledge is power, and with this chapter I'm going to teach you some of the most important principles and physiologic mechanisms involved in your weight management. When you understand these principles, you will know what your body is doing and why things work the way they do, including why most people gain the weight back after a short, vigorous weight loss program. I usually go over this information with my patients during their first weight management consult. It's amazing how responsive they are to this information. I believe that knowledge of these key principles helps people define their weight loss goals. It also helps patients understand some fundamental human physiology and therefore allows them to lose weight the proper way

We will review the following key concepts:

What is a Body Mass Index (BMI)

How a carbohydrate-controlled diet really works

The hormone leptin and its role in weight loss

Body Mass Index (BMI)

Let's start with the Body Mass Index, otherwise known as the BMI. The BMI is how we define obesity. For adults, it is equal to your weight in kilograms divided by your height in meters squared:

$$BMI = \frac{Weight\ (kilograms)}{Height\ (meters)^2}$$

To calculate your weight in kilograms you should check your weight in pounds and then divide that number by 2.2. That will give you your weight in kilograms. Measure your height in centimeters (one inch is equal to 2.54 centimeters) and then divide that number by 100 to get your height in meters. Then, multiply that number by itself to get the height in meters squared. For example:

What is the BMI of a 220 pound person who is 160 cm tall?

220 pounds/2.2 = 100 kg

160 cm/100 = 1.6 meters

1.6 X 1.6 = 2.56 meters squared

BMI = 100/2.56 = 39

Now that we've reviewed the hard way of calculating your BMI, let's review the easy way. Simply refer to the following chart, find your height (inches) and weight (pounds), and you'll have your BMI.

Body Mass Index (BMI) chart

BMI	19	20	21	22	23	24	25	26	27	28	29	30	31	32	33	34	35	36
Ht. (in.)	Body Weight (pounds)																	
58	91	96	100	105	110	115	119	124	129	134	138	143	148	153	158	162	167	172
59	94	99	104	109	114	119	124	128	133	138	143	148	153	158	163	168	173	178
60	97	102	107	112	118	123	128	133	138	143	148	153	158	163	168	174	179	184
61	100	106	111	116	122	127	132	137	143	148	153	158	164	169	174	180	185	190
62	104	109	115	120	126	131	136	142	147	153	158	164	169	175	180	186	191	196
63	107	113	118	124	130	135	141	146	152	158	163	169	175	180	186	191	197	203
64	110	116	122	128	134	140	145	151	157	163	169	174	180	186	192	197	204	209
65	114	120	126	132	138	144	150	156	162	168	174	180	186	192	198	204	210	216
66	118	124	130	136	142	148	155	161	167	173	179	186	192	198	204	210	216	223
67	121	127	134	140	146	153	159	166	172	178	185	191	198	204	211	217	223	230
68	125	131	138	144	151	158	164	171	177	184	190	197	203	210	216	223	230	236
69	128	135	142	149	155	162	169	176	182	189	196	203	209	216	223	230	236	243
70	132	139	146	153	160	167	174	181	188	195	202	209	216	222	229	236	243	250
71	136	143	150	157	165	172	179	186	193	200	208	215	222	229	236	243	250	257
72	140	147	154	162	169	177	184	191	199	206	213	221	228	235	242	250	258	265
73	144	151	159	166	174	182	189	197	204	212	219	227	235	242	250	257	265	272
74	148	155	163	171	179	186	194	202	210	218	225	233	241	249	256	264	272	280
75	152	160	168	176	184	192	200	208	216	224	232	240	248	256	264	272	279	287
76	156	164	172	180	189	197	205	213	221	230	238	246	254	263	271	279	287	295

BMI	37	38	39	40	41	42	43	44	45	46	47	48	49	50	51	52	53	54
Ht. (in.)	Body Weight (pounds)																	
58	177	181	186	191	196	201	205	210	215	220	224	229	234	239	244	248	253	258
59	183	188	193	198	203	208	212	217	222	227	232	237	242	247	252	257	262	267
60	189	194	199	204	209	215	220	225	230	235	240	245	250	255	261	266	271	276
61	195	201	206	211	217	222	227	232	238	243	248	254	259	264	269	275	280	285
62	202	207	213	218	224	229	235	240	246	251	256	262	267	273	278	284	289	295
63	208	214	220	225	231	237	242	248	254	259	265	270	278	282	287	293	299	304
64	215	221	227	232	238	244	250	256	262	267	273	279	285	291	296	302	308	314
65	222	228	234	240	246	252	258	264	270	276	282	288	294	300	306	312	318	324
66	229	235	241	247	253	260	266	272	278	284	291	297	303	309	315	322	328	334
67	236	242	249	255	261	268	274	280	287	293	299	306	312	319	325	331	338	344
68	243	249	256	262	269	276	282	289	295	302	308	315	322	328	335	341	348	354
69	250	257	263	270	277	284	291	297	304	311	318	324	331	338	345	351	358	365
70	257	264	271	278	285	292	299	306	313	320	327	334	341	348	355	362	369	376
71	265	272	279	286	293	301	308	315	322	329	338	343	351	358	365	372	379	386
72	272	279	287	294	302	309	316	324	331	338	346	353	361	368	375	383	390	397
73	280	288	295	302	310	318	325	333	340	348	355	363	371	378	386	393	401	408
74	287	295	303	311	319	326	334	342	350	358	365	373	381	389	396	404	412	420
75	295	303	311	319	327	335	343	351	359	367	375	383	391	399	407	415	423	431
76	304	312	320	328	336	344	353	361	369	377	385	394	402	410	418	426	435	443

Adapted from the NHLBI Obesity guidelines
(http://www.nhlbi.nih.gov/guidelines/obesity/bmi_tbl.htm)

Now, here is how you classify your weight based on your BMI:

BMI	Classification
18.5-20	Normal
25-30	Overweight
30-40	Obese (high risk for many diseases)
> 40	Morbidly Obese (severely high risk)

Our theoretical patient has a BMI of 39 so he fits under the "obese" classification. He is a perfect candidate for the 6-Step Weight Loss program. Why don't you try and calculate your own BMI? Mine is 20.*

*The Body Mass Index equation is well accepted in the medical community as a means of classifying obesity for most adults. It should be noted however, that it is inaccurate for certain populations including pregnant women, children, and body builders. If you fit in one of these categories, you will need to consult your doctor regarding your weight classification.

The Carbohydrate Controlled Diet

Now you know your weight classification. Let's talk a little about the "carb-controlled phenomenon." From a physiologic standpoint, the carb-controlled diet makes a lot of sense and actually works wonderfully for many people. A particular misconception about this style of dieting is that it is something "new." Carb-controlled dieting has been around since the 4th century BC and was actually recommended by Hippocrates himself (father of modern medicine) for his obese pa-

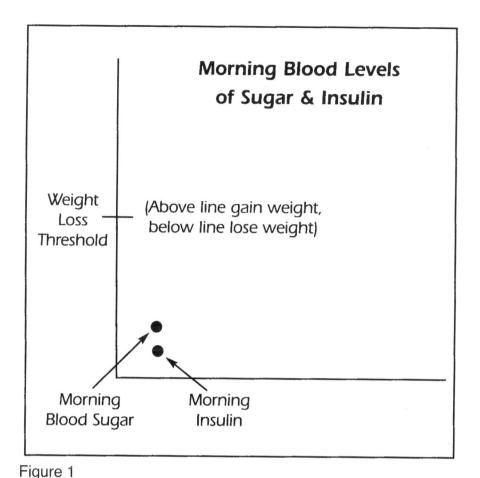

Figure 1

tients (5). Throughout history, certain pioneering individuals re-popularized the idea of carb-controlled weight loss dieting in their respective societies and time periods. These individuals include: the virtually unknown British undertaker William Banting (1797-1876); the German physician Wilhelm Ebstein (1836-1912); and the American cardiologist and diet guru Robert Atkins (1930-2003).

Since its re-popularization in modern times, the concept of carb- controlled dieting has been morphed into a number of popular diet books

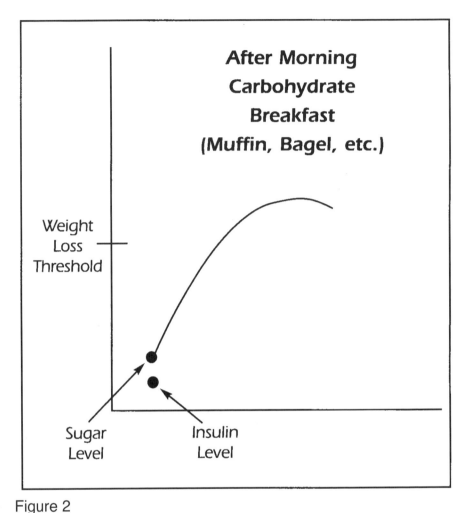

Figure 2

and weight loss publications (some more sophisticated then others). In
addition, many studies have been done at reputable medical institutions
demonstrating the safety and effectiveness of carb-controlled dieting
(6,7). Here is how the carb-controlled diet works.

1. Your pancreas secretes insulin. The pancreas is basically a gland
   sitting in the middle of your back behind your stomach. Insulin
   is responsible for sugar utilization and conversion of extra calo-

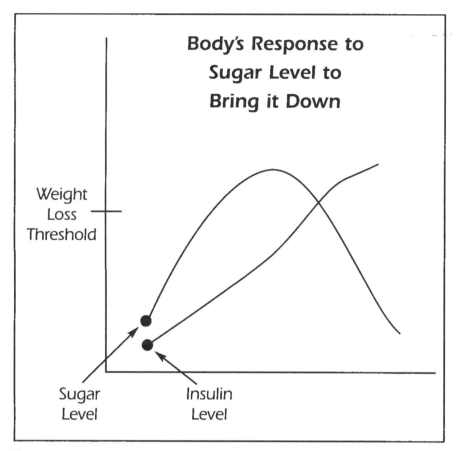

Body's Response to Sugar Level to Bring it Down

Weight Loss Threshold

Sugar Level

Insulin Level

Figure 3

ries into fat molecules. When insulin levels are high, you gain weight.

2. Insulin is secreted by the pancreas in response to the intake of sugars. Sugars and carbohydrates are the same thing. They are synonyms (refer to **Figure 2**).

3. When sugar levels, which are the same thing as carbohydrate levels, go up (like after eating that morning muffin or bagel) your pancreas responds by shooting out insulin to start metabolizing

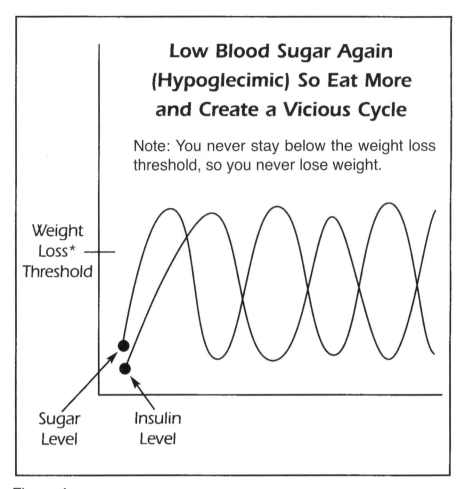

Low Blood Sugar Again (Hypoglecimic) So Eat More and Create a Vicious Cycle

Note: You never stay below the weight loss threshold, so you never lose weight.

Weight Loss* Threshold

Sugar Level

Insulin Level

Figure 4

that sugar and to help produce fat molecules to store it (**Figures 3 and 4**).

4. As a result, the now high insulin levels cause your body to become hypoglycemic (low-sugar). The rapid rise in insulin has caused the sugar to move from the blood into different cells, including fat cells for fat production, so your blood sugar level is now low again (**Figure 4**).

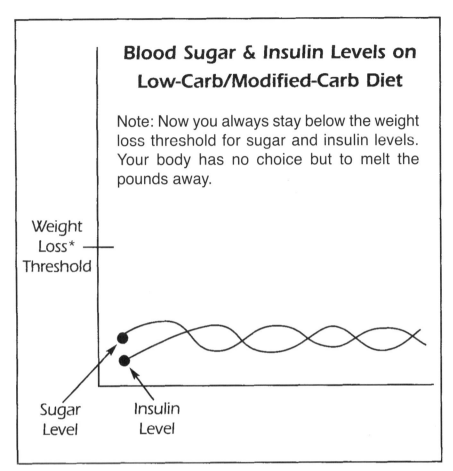

Blood Sugar & Insulin Levels on Low-Carb/Modified-Carb Diet

Note: Now you always stay below the weight loss threshold for sugar and insulin levels. Your body has no choice but to melt the pounds away.

Weight Loss* Threshold

Sugar Level

Insulin Level

Figure 5

5. Your hypothalamus (which is the part of the brain responsible for appetite control) now senses the low blood sugar and tells your body that you are hungry again.

6. You are now hungry again and eat more either to gain weight or stay the same. This is a vicious cycle that happens throughout the day (**Figure 5**). Remember how you are always hungry one to two hours after eating Chinese food, which is very rich in car-

bohydrates like noodles, rice, sweet sauces, etc. Well, this is what's going on.

Now consider the carb-controlled diet. Notice how the lines stay well below the weight threshold line. Your body has no choice but to melt the fat away and lose the weight.

The 6-Step Weight Loss Diet (discussed in detail in the next chapter) is a type of carb-controlled diet. However, we are unique from other carb-controlled diets in that we utilize a proprietary *multi-dimensional nutritional analysis* technique to categorize various foods in our diet. This technique takes into consideration not only the nutritional facts of a particular food, but also many other factors of the food which may influence weight loss including: ingredients, portion controlled serving size, surface area to volume ratio of food particles (for certain foods), glycemic load, food availability, brand specification, and taste appeal. We believe this technique has been one of the key components to the enormous success our patients have had. I'll explain the details of our *multi-dimensional nutritional analysis technique* in the next chapter.

The Role of Leptin

Now we will discuss the role of the hormone leptin in body weight regulation. This is crucial to understanding not so much the weight loss component of the program, but the weight loss maintenance.

Your fat cells secrete a neurohormone called leptin, which acts on r so. It has been clinically proven that overweight patients who lose as little as 10% of their weight have a significant reduction in the risk of developing many serious medical illnesses including coronary heart disease and diabetes.(10,11) Even if you do not reach your ideal body weight, BMI between 20 to 25, by losing 10% of weight you gain a significant health benefit.

Once that first goal of 10% of weight loss is achieved we reset our goals to a cruise control mode. All efforts at "weight loss" are ceased and diverted exclusively to "weight maintenance." This is a crucial part of the process and it is how we deal with the influence of leptin. We stay in this phase for about 8-12 weeks. During this time, your hypothalamus will get used to the lower concentration of leptin. It now resets its receptors for the leptin hormone to the new lower level. Your body then accepts your new lower weight as normal and stops that initial powerful force trying to bring you back to your old weight. This is a theoretical model that I feel must be dealt with for any weight management program to be successful. After that 8-12 week weight maintenance phase, we go back to weight loss again if needed. Slow and steady wins the race. Weight management is no different.

You now understand some fundamental principles of weight classification and weight management on the scientific level. This understanding is crucial to your success. Sometimes the medical language can be burdensome. I've tried to simplify the explanations as the best I could. If you did not understand some parts of the previous discussion please go back and reread those parts. This book is quite short so it shouldn't take you long to do so.

Knowledge is power, and now you are empowered to move on to Step 3! Let's review The 6-Step Diet.

Step 3:
6-Step Weight Loss Diet

I n the previous edition of this book, I advocated an approach involving individual diet selection: matching the right diet with the right person. I still believe that weight loss can never follow a "cookie-cutter" formula and that the individualized approach to weight loss works best for the greatest number of people. Not everyone wears a size "9-D" shoe; therefore, not everyone will require the exact same intervention to obtain weight loss success. There are a number of reasonably good diets available (some better than others), and if you personally have achieved success on a particular one then maybe that one is best for you. You can use the other principles in this book to help you understand how best to keep the weight off.

However, if you've been frustrated time and time again with weight loss or weight loss maintenance failure, then I highly encourage you to pay especially close attention to this chapter. I'm going to review for you in detail the 6-Step Weight Loss Diet. We'll also review how we utilize our proprietary *multi-dimensional nutritional analysis* technique to turn weight loss into "an 80% knowledge and 20% effort" experience. Let's get started.

The 6-Step Weight Loss Diet has been designed to enhance your fat burning hormones and minimize your fat storing hormones. By eating the *right* foods and taking the *right* nutritional supplement you do have control of these hormones. The body is a complicated structure and there are literally dozens of different hormones and neurotransmitters involved in weight regulation (Figure 1). With the 6-Step Weight Loss Diet you are going to take advantage of years of scientific research in this field to give you the absolute greatest chance for successful weight loss. The diet is a physiologic diet which means it works *with*, not against, your natural body functions to achieve and sustain healthy weight loss.

Figure 1: Various hormones involved in body weight regulation

insulin	CART
leptin	growth hormone
Ghrelin	cortisol
neuropeptide Y	DHEA
CCK	thyroid hormone
resistin	testosterone
adiponectin	estrogen
progesterone	MSH
MCH	PPY

The 6-Step Weight Loss Diet

Take Control of Your Fat Burning Hormones

Category 1 (unlimited)

-all vegetables in abundance (except potatoes, squash, corn, and carrots)
-legumes (including beans and lentils)
-fish (any and all types including shellfish, cooked any way but deep fried)
-lean cuts of beef, veal, and lamb
-skinless chicken and turkey
-tuna salad and chicken salad (made with low-fat mayo only)
-low-fat lunch meat
-low-fat cheese and cheese sticks
-hummus (Mediterranean ground chick peas)
-eggs (fried, scrambled, boiled, omlette)
-olive oil cooking spray (for pan frying, no deep frying allowed)
-sugar-free jell-O,
-*6-Step Weight Loss* Soup Mixes (Chicken, Beef Vegetable*)*
-*6-Step Weight Loss* Shakes (Chocolate or Vanilla)

Condiments:

-low-fat blended butter (*Smart Balance*® Butter Light preferred, no margarine)
-low-fat mayo (any brand)
-sugar free or low-carb ketchup (*Heinz*® One Carb brand preferred)
-low-calorie salad dressing (*Maple Grove Farms*® Sugar Free Balsalmic or Rasberry
  Vinagrette, *South Beach Diet*® Ranch, *Ken's Steak House*® Lite Ceasar, *Wishbone*®
  Salad Spritzer Italian or Balsamic Breeze preferred)
-mustard (any brand, no honey-mustard)
-pickles (includes relish, no sweet pickles or sweet relish)
-all powdered spices (salt, pepper, oregano, basil, tumeric, saffron, curry powder.......)
-sugar free jelly (*Fifty50*® Sugar Free-Low Calorie Jelly any flavor)

Beverages:

-water in abundance
-diet caffeine free soda
-diet ice teas (including *Crystal Light®,* diet *Snapple®,* diet *Arizona®…*)
-diet fruit drinks (including *Minute Made® Light* and *Tropicana® Sugar
	Free* drinks)
-decaf coffee (any brand, may use non-dairy creamer and/or no-calorie
	sweetener)
-*6-StepWeight Loss*™ fiber mixed fruit drink

Category 2 (two servings per day)

-apple (medium sized with the peel)
-pear (medium sized with the peel)
-strawberries (1 cup)
-raspberries (1 cup)
-blueberries (1 cup)
-blackberries (1 cup)
-grapefruit (medium sized)
-cantaloupe (1 cup cubed)
-whole wheat bread (1 slice is a serving. Should be less than 50 calories per
	slice and
  have at least 3 grams of fiber per slice-we recommend *Nature's Own®* dou-
	ble fiber or
  Nature's Own® wheat & fiber)
-low-carb tortilla wrap (1 wrap is a serving, any brand)
-1% low-fat or skim milk (1 cup)
-low-fat yogurt (one 4 oz cup and should have no sugar added)
-whole wheat pasta (1/2 cup cooked)
-peanut butter (two tablespoons, any brand except for brands that say "low-
	fat")
-Nuts (twenty only, of any kind including: peanuts, walnuts, cashew nuts,…)
-*6-Step Weight Loss* Classic Oatmeal (this is the only oatmeal allowed on
	diet)
-*6-Step Weight Loss* Pancakes with syrup (one package)
-*6-Step Weight Loss* Honey Nut Flavored Soy Cereals

Category 3 (forbidden)

-regular fruit juices
-white bread
-rice (of any kind including brown rice and wild rice)
-french fries
-potato chips
-candy bars
-potatoes
-white pasta
-regular soda
-margarine
-regular ketchup
-table sugar
-popcorn (of any kind, including low-fat)
-alcohol

Category 4 (2 servings per day)

-*6-Step Weight Loss* Fudge Graham Bar
-*6-Step Weight Loss* Chocolate Peanut Bar,
-*6-Step Weight Loss* Cinammon Bar
-*6-Step Weight Loss* Pretzel Mix
-*6-Step Weight Loss* Chocolate Cereal Bar
-*6-Step Weight Loss* Caramel Cereal Bar
-*6-Step Weight Loss* Soy Nut Mix
-*Breyers*® Carb Smart Ice Cream Almond Bar
-*Breyers*® Carb Smart Ice Cream Fudge Bar
-*Lindt*® 70% Dark Chocolate (1/3 of 100g bar)

Instructions for 6-Step Weight Loss Diet

Category 1 Foods:

This is the category of foods you can eat in abundance. No weighing, measuring, or note taking of calories! You should eat until satisfied but don't overstuff yourself. Your stomach is only the size of your fist. Regarding the vegetables, I would like you to focus your intake on vegetables you would normally find in a salad (ie, lettuce, cucumbers, broccoli, tomatoes, etc.); however, other vegetables like legumes and beans are also permissible. Avoid potatoes, corn, squash, and carrots as stated since these vegetables are very glycemic and stimulate elevated insulin levels.

Try and eat fresh, lean meats including poultry, beef, veal, lamb and fish. Fresh, unprocessed meat contains higher levels of naturally occurring conjugated linoleic acid (CLA) which supports the fat burning process. Processed meats including low fat lunch meats are permissible; however, when given the choice, go for the fresh meat.

Eggs are a great source of protein during weight loss. They are filled with many essential nutrients including the essential amino acid lysine, which helps protect lean muscle mass during weight loss. Egg protein has the highest biological value compared to any other protein source. If you have high cholesterol you may use egg whites instead. Use olive oil cooking spray when frying eggs or other foods from this category.

Category 2 Foods:

This is your restricted category. You may have up to two servings of anything on this list per day, but only two. Notice that the serving size is included next to most of the items. You should mix and match in this category to help keep things interesting. There is no time restriction for when you can have these foods. In other words, it is fine to eat them during the morning, afternoon, and evening. The only restriction is the two-serving daily limit.

For example, maybe one day you will choose a slice of whole wheat bread along with a serving (two tablespoons) of peanut butter.

Then you're done for the day. Maybe another day you will choose to have an apple (medium sized) and a cup of low fat milk. Then you're done. Another day you may have a half cup whole wheat pasta and a handful of nuts (twenty). You get the point. Pretty straightforward.

Category 3 Foods:

These are the forbidden foods! They are filled with macronutrients that stimulate high levels of fat storing hormones and inhibit fat burning hormones. You will want to empty your pantry/refrigerator of all these foods to help you avoid them during your weight loss phase. Once you have been off these foods for the first week or so, avoiding them will become much easier. We can bring back some of these foods in moderation during your weight maintenance cycle, but for the time being (during a weight loss cycle) they are off limits. I am often asked why alcohol is forbidden during the weight loss cycle of the diet. Alcohol stimulates a specific receptor on fat cells called alpha receptors. When stimulated, alpha receptors signal the fat cell to store excess energy as fat, instead of burning it off as fuel. For this reason alcohol can often slow down weight loss. We'll discuss the 6-Step Weight Maintenance Diet in further detail and how to bring back some of the Category 3 foods back into the diet in the weight loss maintenance chapter.

Category 4 foods:

These are the allowable snack foods on the diet. A lot of effort has gone into developing this section; so stick to it closely! Try to avoid the low-carb blitz currently going on in the diet and food industry. Many of these food products do not have sufficient fiber or protein content which help to manage long-term hunger. In addition, many contain a high dose of sugar alcohols which tend to be glycemic and are very poor at satisfying the appetite, leading to an increase, not decrease, in calorie intake. For these reasons, our center has developed a number of products in this category which are high in fiber, high in quality protein, low glycemic, and taste delicious. For **6-Step Weight Loss** distributed items you can visit www.6stepweightloss.com. Otherwise, a number of these products you should be able to find in your local grocery store.

There is a restriction of only two items from this list per day, with one exception.

If you use any of the Category 4 items to replace a meal (breakfast, lunch, or dinner) that does not count against your two item quota for the day. For example, if you decide one morning to have a *6-Step Weight Loss* Fudge Graham Bar in place of breakfast, you still have two more Category 4 items left to eat for that day. Another day, if you are not feeling very hungry in the afternoon and decide to have a bar in place of lunch, then you still have two Category 4 items left for the day..... Feel free to make this substitution as often, or in often as you like.

Nutritional Supplementation:

1) You must drink at least 64 oz of water and take a multivitamin every day. We highly recommend the *6-Step Essentials*. The 6-Step Essentials has been exclusively designed for Dr. Virji's 6-Step Weight Loss program. The supplement is rich in the most common vitamins deficient in the average American diet including Zinc, Magnesium, Vitamin B-6, Vitamin C, Folate, and Thiamin (12). In addition, we have added sufficient doses of Calcium, Chromium, Vanadium, and Carnitine to further support healthy weight. Calcium supplementation has been clinically proven to inhibit intracellular fat storing enzymes (13). The calcium has been sufficiently balanced with magnesium to support overall cardiovascular health. Chromium and Vanadium have shown benefits in weight loss through their potential effect on helping to regulate the body's insulin function (14). We have added only the purist form of L-Carnitine to help support the body's fat burning capacity which may also help to increase energy levels during weight loss (15). The 6-Step Essentials supplement has been intelligently designed to support healthy weight in the context of sustaining overall health. They can be found at www.6-stepweightloss.com.

2) You must take a dietary fiber supplement, 2 tablespoons in a full glass of water (or a sugar-free, non-carbonated drink of your choice) with breakfast and dinner every day. I recommend guar gum as your fiber supplement because in addition to its benefits of reducing risk of colon cancer and keeping you regular (benefits of most dietary fiber supplements), guar gum has the added benefit

of natural appetite suppression.* Guar gum works like a sponge in the stomach to reduce the appetite by stimulating stomach stretch receptors as well as lowers the glycemic index of the other foods eaten. A popular over-the-counter brand of fiber supplement recently replaced guar gum as its main ingredient with another type of fiber called wheat dextrin. Because my patients were finding it difficult to find guar gum over-the-counter, our center developed its own brand of fiber drink with guar gum to ensure patients had access to it. The *6-Step Weight Loss* Fiber mixed fruit drink (one packet in a full glass of water twice daily) will fulfill your daily dietary fiber requirement in a very tasty way (tastes like Koolaid)! Other common brands of dietary fiber include psillium husk (*Metamucil®)* and Methylcellulose (*Citrucel®)*. These can be found in your local grocery store and can be used as an option only if you can't find guar gum and are unable to use our brand.

*Two things should be noted about guar gum though. The first is that guar gum won't help you lose weight unless its use is part of a greater weight management program.(15) The second is that in the past, manufacturers of certain herbal weight loss medications utilized very high concentrations of guar gum in their supplements. This super-high concentration of guar gum led to a number of cases of gastrointestinal obstruction in people using them. The FDA has since banned its use in such high concentrations in weight loss pills. It is still routinely used as a food thickener, stool softener, and dietary fiber supplement.

Advantages of The 6-Step Weight Loss Diet
(What's going on hormonally in your body)

1) Low in simple and complex sugar: This aspect of the plan helps to reduce the body's insulin levels. Elevated insulin not only supports fat storage in the body, but also increases your risk for cardiovascular disease (16). This is a state known as "Insulin Resistance."

2) Increased beneficial proteins: This aspect of the plan stimulates postprandial thermogenesis (your body's metabolism after eating) and increases the body's glucagon level (17). Glucagon is another hormone produced by your body's pancreas which pro-

motes healthy fat burning working at the opposite level of insulin. You want these levels high.

3) Low in caffeine: This aspect of the plan prevents inhibition of your body's growth hormone release. (18) Growth hormone is important in helping your body hold on to lean muscle during weight loss. Remember, you want to lose the fat cells not the muscle. Getting a regular good night's sleep is also helpful in promoting healthy growth hormone levels.

4) High in Omega 3 FA: (from such items as fish, olive oil, and nuts) stimulates an enzyme called CPT (Carnitine Palmotyl Transferase) to increase the body's carnitine level. Carnitine supports fat burning and energy level during weight loss. (19) There is also added carnitine to the 6-Step Essentials vitamin supplement to further enhance this effect.

5) Calcium: (from such items as cheese, low-fat dairy products, and green leafy vegetables) This inhibits an enzyme called Fatty Acid Synthetase inside fat cells to help prevent fat synthesis and production (20). The 6-Step Essentials is also fortified with calcium and balanced with magnesium for optimal nutrition.

6) Guar gum: This is a type of dietary fiber that is supplemented in the diet. Guar gum helps reduce the glycemic index of the foods you eat as well as increases a sense of fullness after meals, acting as an all-natural appetite suppressant (21).

7) Phytochemicals: (from the variety of different vegetables allowed on the plan) When consumed in abundance they reduce your risk of cardiovascular disease as well as potentially reduce your risk for certain types of cancer (22).

Sample Menus

Day One:

Breakfast:
6-Step Essentials Nutritional Weight Loss Supplement
6-Step Weight Loss© Fiber Fulfill mixed fruit drink
Western Style Omelet with onions, green peppers, and cheese
1 slice of whole wheat bread (*Nature's Own*® Double Fiber recommended)
Sugar free ice tea and/or cup of decaf coffee

Snack:
Medium sized apple (eaten with the peel)

Lunch:
Terriaki Grouper with mixed vegetables
Side salad
Diet caffeine free soda

Snack:
6-Step Weight Loss Fudge Graham Bar

Dinner:
6-Step Weight Loss Fiber Fulfill mixed fruit drink
Petite Sirloin Steak with steamed broccoli and mashed cauliflower
(available at *Ruby Tuesdays*® Restaurant)
Diet Caffeine free soda or sugar free ice tea

Dessert:
6-Step Weight Loss© Chocolate Peanut Bar

Category Calculator
Two Category 2's (slice of bread and apple)
Two Category 4's (6-Step Fudge Graham Bar and Chocolate Peanut Bar)

* Make sure to get in 64 oz of water (that's eight 8-ounce glasses a day)

Day Two:

Breakfast:
6-Step Essentials Nutritional Weight Loss Supplement
6-Step Weight Loss Fiber Fulfill mixed fruit drink
2 Slices of turkey bacon
Scrambled eggs
Sugar free ice tea and/or cup of decaf coffee

Snack:
Cup of strawberries

Lunch:
Cup of tuna or chicken salad
One slice of Whole wheat bread
Sugar free jello

Snack:
6-Step Weight Loss Chocolate Peanut Bar

Dinner:
6-Step Weight Loss Fiber Fulfill mixed fruit drink
Greek gyro platter
Side of hummus and Greek salad

Dessert:
Breyers® Carb Smart Ice Cream Almond Bar

Category Calculator
Two Category 2's (cup of strawberries and slice of bread)
Two Category 4's (6-Step Chocolate Peanut Bar and Breyer's Ice Cream
    Almond Bar)

* Make sure to get in 64 oz of water (that's eight 8-ounce glasses a day)

Day Three:

Breakfast:
6-Step Essentials Nutritional Weight Loss Supplement
6-Step Weight Loss Fiber Fulfill mixed fruit drink
6-Step Weight Loss maple brown sugar oatmeal
Medium sized pear with the peel

Snack:
6-StepWeight Loss Cinnamon Bar

Lunch:
Mixed Grill with steamed broccoli and Caesar salad (no croutons)
(Available at *The Olive Garden* Restaurant)
Diet ice tea

Snack:
Sugar free jello

Dinner:
6-Step Weight Loss Fiber Fulfill mixed fruit drink
Prime rib with assorted vegetables
Side salad
Diet caffeine free soda

Dessert:
6-Step Weight Loss Fudge Graham Bar

Category Calculator
Two Category 2's (6-Step Oatmeal and pear)
Two Category 4's (6-Step Cinnamon Bar and Fudge Graham Bar)

* Make sure to get in 64 oz of water (that's eight 8-ounce glasses a day)

Day Four:

Breakfast:
6-Step Essentials Nutritional Weight Loss Supplement
6-Step Weight Loss Fiber Fulfill mixed fruit drink
6-Step Weight Loss maple brown sugar oatmeal
One cup of decaf coffee

Snack:
Low-fat cheese stick

Lunch:
Subway® turkey sub on their low-carb wrap (with any desired toppings)
Diet caffeine free soda

Snack:
6-Step Weight Loss Fudge Graham Bar

Dinner:
6-Step Weight Loss Fiber Fulfill mixed fruit drink
Rotisserie chicken with green beans and side salad
Diet Caffeine free soda or sugar free ice tea

Dessert:
6-Step Weight Loss© Chocolate Peanut Bar

Category Calculator
Two Category 2's (6-Step Oatmeal and low-carb wrap)
Two Category 4's (6-Step Fudge Graham Bar and Chocolate Peanut Bar)

* Make sure to get in 64 oz of water (that's eight 8-ounce glasses a day)

Day Five:

Breakfast:
6-Step Essentials Nutritional Weight Loss Supplement
6-Step Weight Loss Fiber Fulfill mixed fruit drink
6-Step Weight Loss Pancakes with syrup
One cup of 1% low fat or skim milk

Snack:
Low-fat cheese stick

Lunch:
Buffalo chicken salad (available at *TGI Fridays®*)
Diet caffeine free soda

Snack:
6-Step Weight Loss Cocoa Café Bar

Dinner:
6-Step Weight Loss Fiber Fulfill mixed fruit drink
Eggplant Rollette (see section on 6-Step Recipes)
Tossed salad
Diet Caffeine free soda

Dessert:
Lindt® 70% Dark Chocolate (1/3 of the 100g bar)

<u>Category Calculator</u>
Two Category 2's (6-Step Pancake and skim milk)
Two Category 4's (6-Step Cocoa Cafe Bar and Lindt Dark Chocolate)

* Make sure to get in 64 oz of water (that's eight 8-ounce glasses a day)

Day Six:

Breakfast:
6-Step Essentials Nutritional Weight Loss Supplement
6-Step Weight Loss Fiber mixed fruit drink
6-Step Weight Loss Fudge Graham Bar

Snack:
1 cup of cantaloupe

Lunch:
South Beach Diet® Chicken Caesar Wraps (1 box)
Diet caffeine free soda

Snack:
6-Step Weight Loss Cinnamon Bar

Dinner:
6-Step Weight Loss Fiber Fulfill mixed fruit drink
Spicy Lemon Grilled chicken (see section on 6-Step Recipes)
6-Step Weight Loss Beef Vegetable Soup
Diet ice tea

Dessert:
Breyers® Carb Smart Ice Cream Almond Bar

Category Calculator
Two Category 2's (1 cup cantaloupe and South Beach Diet Chicken Cae-
    sar Wrap)
Two Category 4's (6-Step Cinnamon Bar and Breyers Ice Cream Almond
    Bar)
(6-Step Fudge Graham Bar was used as a meal replacement so doesn't
    count!)

* Make sure to get in 64 oz of water (that's eight 8-ounce glasses a day)

Day Seven:

Breakfast:
6-Step Essentials Nutritional Weight Loss Supplement
6-Step Weight Loss Fiber mixed fruit drink
Homemade Tuna Salad (made with low fat mayo)
1 slice of whole wheat bread (*Nature's Own*® Double Fiber recommended)
1 cup of decaf coffee

Snack:
1 cup of low-fat yogurt (no sugar added)

Lunch:
6-Step Weight Loss Chicken Noodle Soup
Diet caffeine free soda

Snack:
6-Step Weight Loss Fudge Graham Bar

Dinner:
6-Step Weight Loss Fiber Fulfill mixed fruit drink
Authentic Italian Ministrone Soup (see section on 6-Step Recipes)
Diet ice tea

Dessert:
Breyers® Carb Smart Ice Cream Almond Bar

Category Calculator
Two Cátegory 2's (slice of bread and low-fat yogurt)
Two Category 4's (6-Step Fudge Graham Bar and Breyer's Ice Cream AlmondBar)

* Make sure to get in 64 oz of water (that's eight 8-ounce glasses a day)

Multi-dimensional Nutritional Analysis Technique

Nutritional Information: This is the first aspect of a particular food we take into consideration before placing it on our diet. In general, a particular food is made up of four major nutrients: carbohydrate, protein, fat, and water. These nutrients play a vital role in determining the calorie content of food (*energy density*). In addition, they play a vital role in determining your body and your metabolism's reaction to the food (*thermogenesis*). Ideally, you want to consume foods that are low in *energy density,* but that are high in *thermogenicity.* This is very important to understand!

Let's briefly consider the traditional low-fat diet and the traditional low-carb diet to better understand how the 6-Step Weight Loss Diet approach differs. Low-fat diets emphasize the reduction in the intake of dietary fats. Dietary fat, in and of itself, is highly *energy dense* and therefore contains a large number of calories per gram. By reducing fat intake and by tracking calories, a low-fat diet helps you lose weight by reducing total calorie intake. You are generally recommended to eat more fruits and vegetables and avoid foods high in fat. There are a few problems I see with this approach to dieting.

Firstly, although a low-fat diet is low in *energy density* (which is good), it does nothing to help control your appetite and rev up your body's metabolism. So, a low-fat diet is poorly *thermogenic.* Dietary fat is primarily replaced by dietary carbohydrate on a traditional low-fat diet. Your body can easily break down and store dietary carbohydrate as fat without using much energy in the process. In addition, the excess carbohydrate stimulates the secretion of various fat storing hormones including insulin and cortisol thereby sending signals to the body to hold on to excess weight. The insulin also reduces blood sugar which in turn stimulates appetite and causes you to crave more food (see figure 2-5 in previous chapter). Ever wonder why you were always so hungry while on a low fat diet in the past? Excess dietary carbohydrate, particularly refined carbohydrate, reduces levels of certain fat burning hormones in the body including glucagon and growth hormone, making it even harder to lose weight on a traditional low-fat diet.

Secondly, the simple recommendation to "eat more fruits and vegetables" is too vague to help with actual weight loss. Which fruits? Which vegetables? Sugar cane (where table sugar comes from) is a vegetable. French fries and ketchup are two vegetables. You obviously wouldn't recommend someone eat more sugar cane, french fries, and ketchup to lose weight. It is important to know which fruits and vegetables not only contain the least amount of calories but also are the least insulin stimulating. For example, a cup of blueberries is high in fiber, low in sugar, and low in calories. A cup of watermelon is low in fiber, high in sugar, and high in calories. They are obviously both fruits, but they each have very different effects on the body when consumed. The recommendation to "eat more fruits and vegetables" because they are low in fat is not well-founded. You need to further break down the various fruits and vegetables into those that help sustain weight loss and those that do not. In Category 1 and 2 of the 6-Step Diet we have outlined for you the best fruits and vegetables to consume.

Thirdly, not all dietary fat is bad. Strictly consuming a traditional low fat diet may put you at risk for deficiency of good dietary fat. This is a category of dietary fats which we call *essential fats*, meaning the body cannot make them and therefore requires dietary consumption. The two essential dietary fats are *linolenic acid* and *linoleic acid*. *Linolenic acid* is an Omega 3 fatty acid and is commonly found in cold water fish, olive oil, and nuts. *Linoleic acid* is an Omega 6 fatty acid found primarily in plants and vegetable oils. Both of these are considered unsaturated fats and are an essential part of any healthy diet. The ideal ratio of Omega 3 to Omega 6 consumption in the diet is 1:4. The current Western Diet is unbalanced at a 1:20 ratio.

These fats play a crucial role in a number of the body's physiologic functions. Eighty percent of the brain and central nervous system is made from these fats, known as the *white matter* of the brain. Studies which have replaced dietary carbohydrate with unsaturated fat have led to significant improvements in good cholesterol and triglyceride levels (28). In addition, many of our body's hormones come from dietary fat building blocks, including estrogen in women and testosterone in men.

It is true that any type of dietary fat (including monounsaturated, polyunsaturated, saturated, and trans fats) is more energy dense than carbohydrate and protein. But to recommend the consumption of a low-fat diet is minimalistic in my opinion and not helpful for overall weight loss or overall health. Instead, we should focus on consuming a diet low in trans fat and saturated fat (the bad fats) while also being mindful of energy density.

In summary, the traditional low-fat diet is low in *energy density,* but is poorly *thermogenic.* So it provides us with only one half of the solution to a successful weight loss diet. Let's take a look at the other half of the solution and consider the traditional low-carb diet.

The traditional low-carb diet is a type of qualitative carb-controlled diet that involves the limited consumption of dietary carbohydrates to stimulate ketosis and fat burning. In the previous chapter, I've described in detail how this style of dieting can reduce insulin levels and other fat storing hormones while simultaneously helping you to control appetite. In addition, the increased consumption of dietary protein increases the amount of work the body has to do to digest meals. Hence, the body has to burn more calories to digest the food and a feeling of fullness tends to last longer. This is called *post-prandial thermogensis* and is another strength of the low-carb approach to dieting. For the above reasons, a low-carb diet tends to be highly *thermogenic.* Unfortunately, because of the poor regulation of dietary fat and calorie intake it tends to also be highly *energy dense.*

In addition, many food companies have substituted sugar in their "low-carb" foods with sugar alcohols (maltilol, sorbitol, xylitol) thereby keeping the "net carbs" low but "net calories" still high. Sugar alcohols are poorly absorbed sugars that contain about 2.7 calories/gram. Consuming sugar alcohols is better for the body than consuming table sugar, but their consumption still needs to be properly regulated. They are still glycemic meaning that they stimulate insulin secretion and are not very good at quenching the appetite (which may even lead to increased calorie intake in the long run).

Many "low carb" foods are filled with saturated fats, some even with trans fats, which contributes to the high *energy density* of the diet in general. When seeking to lose weight, you have to consider all nutrient constituents in food (protein, carbohydrate, fat, and water) as well as total calories before you can be given free reign to eat it. We have taken this into careful consideration in designing Category 1 of the 6-Step Diet.

The 6-Step Weight Loss Diet is a low *energy dense* and highly *thermogenic* diet. By carefully controlling not only the calories but also the ratio of the various nutrients found in food, you can significantly reduce calorie intake and at the same time rev up your body's metabolism for fat burning and appetite control. It combines the strengths of a low-fat diet (low *energy* density) with the strengths of a low-carb diet (highly *thermogenic*) to help maximize weight loss success. For this reason, you will see low-fat items recommended on the diet at times, and you will see low-carb items recommended at other times. The 6-Step Diet has been designed to make calorie regulation and fat burning significantly easier. On the diet you will find that you do not need to "count" calories to "control" calories. You will maximize your fat burning hormones and minimize your fat storing hormones and effectively control appetite in the process.

The formula we use to accomplish this is quite complex but has been significantly simplified for you by breaking down foods into four specific categories. You just watch your categories, and we'll do the rest of the work! Essentially we have five major nutritional criteria we look at to help us determine which category a particular food will be placed. These criteria include: total calories, total calories/carbohydrate calories ratio; carbohydrate/fiber ratio, total protein, total fat/saturated fat ratio, and total trans fat.

Ingredients: This is the second most important when a food item is considered for placement on the **6-Step Diet**. Unfortunately, the nutritional information found in the little white box on food packaging can be misleading when used alone. The ingredients section gives us valuable information on particular nutrient sources which may play an important role in helping with weight loss.

Let's take the example of protein. Not all protein is created equal! There are many different types of protein out there including: egg, casein, soy, whey, etc. Each protein has its own unique biological value. Biological value refers to the body's ability to use the protein as a building block for body maintenance. That which doesn't get used by the body for routine maintenance gets filtered to the liver and converted to glucose for energy. In general, the higher the biological value of the protein, the higher quality the protein. Egg protein has the highest known biological value that I am aware of (biological value of 48%).

In addition, the quality of a particular protein is also a function of its amino acid composition. Amino acids are the building blocks of proteins, and essential amino acids are those that the body cannot create itself and is therefore reliant on dietary consumption (just like the essential fatty acids). In general, you want to consume proteins that are high in essential amino acids. Egg protein and casein protein are very high in essential amino acids.

Proteins also vary by their insulin index. The insulin index is the ability of a non-carbohydrate containing food to stimulate insulin secretion. Since elevated insulin levels is something we are fighting against when trying to lose weight, you should consume proteins with a lower insulin index. For example, Casein protein (low insulin index) is much better to consume than whey protein (high insulin index) when trying to lose weight. Whey protein is better for muscle building. Special attention to food ingredients and their variable effects on weight loss are taken into consideration when categorizing food in the 6-Step Weight Loss Diet.

Portion Controlled Serving Size: Believe it or not, the amount of food that is placed in front of you during a meal or snack has a large influence on not only your total calorie consumption but also on your feeling of fullness (29). For this reason, foods that have appropriate portion controlled serving sizes are more desireable to consume when trying to lose weight. *This is critical to understand; please pay close attention to the next few paragraphs!*

Let's start out with a few definitions. It is important to understand the difference between "portion size" and "serving size" in order to grasp this very important part of the diet. A portion size is defined as the quantity of food or beverage that an individual selects for consumption. For example, if you are grabbing some french fries at a buffet, the amount that you take off the tray and put in your plate is your portion size. You selected it on your own; it was not served to you. On the other hand, a serving size is defined as a pre-determined quantity of food or beverage that a separate provider selects for an individual's consumption. For example, if you are at a restaurant and you order the sirloin steak and shrimp, your waiter will bring you the serving size of food that the restaurant (separate provider) has determined for you.

It is critical to understand and to accept that your portion size (the amount of food you choose to eat) is greatly affected by your serving size (the amount of food placed in front of you)!

People tend to consume food in units (one cookie, one sandwich, one candy bar, etc.), not in actual weights. In fact, numerous studies have shown that when people are given different serving sizes of the same food on variable days of the week, their portions and hence calorie consumption is directly related to the serving size put in front of them. One study showed that adults served different amounts of macaroni and cheese on different days ate 30% more when given a larger serving size even though there was no difference in their feelings of fullness after the meal. In another study, patients who were served different snack sizes of potato chips before dinner ate up to 37% more calories when served the larger size. More importantly, when dinner came around they did not adjust their food intake to compensate for the increase in snack calories (29).

This phenomenon of serving size controlling portion size has been vigoursly studied in the scientific literature. There exist dozens of studies demonstrating that this is a consistent pattern of human behaviour when it comes to food intake.

Glycemic Index: The glycemic index (GI) of a particular food is basically a measure of the amount of insulin stimulation in the body that results from consumption of that particular food. Since we know that elevated insulin levels lead to appetite stimulation and fat production, foods with the lowest glycemic index are the most desirable. Foods such as rice, potatoes, white bread, and desserts have a very high glycemic index and are avoided in the 6-Step Diet. Foods such as legumes, low-fat cheese, broccoli, lettuce, and cauliflower have a low glycemic index and can be consumed freely in the diet.

One caution with the glycemic index is that it should *not* be overly utilized when developing a dieting strategy. The glycemic index is helpful when used as a tool to classify naturally occurring carbohydrate foods such as fruits, vegetables, legumes, and grains. However, it is not helpful in guiding consumption of processed foods or mixed foods in general. The reason for this is that any particular food item can have its glycemic index lowered by adding fat or protein. The added fat or protein delays the insulin response but often leads to an imbalanced consumption of excess calories. In this situation, the glycemic index of the particular food or meal becomes unimportant when compared to the increased calories and energy density of the food. For example, Peanut *M&M's*® candy and lasagna both have a low glycemic index because of the added fat. Obviously, you will not much lose weight if you load up on either of these two!

Certain diets on the market claim themselves to be *low GI* diets and base almost their entire eating strategy on the glycemic index. This is a misguided approach, in my opinion, and can lead to poor weight loss outcomes. The glycemic index is simply *one* tool in the grand scheme of overall nutritional analysis. When used appropriately it may aid in sustainable weight loss. However, it should not be overly relied upon, particularly when classifying mixed or processed foods.

Food Availability and Brand Specification: In order for a particular dietary strategy to be successful, it must also be practical. In other words, the recommendations made for food consumption should take into consideration available foods and cultural norms of food intake. Adopting abstract recommendations based on geometrical figures (ie, food pyramid) is not a practical way to educate a population on how to lose weight nor on how to eat sensibly in general.

For example, telling an individual to get 60% of calories from carbohydrates, 25% from fat, and 15% from protein is unrealistic (not to mention completely inaccurate and not scientifically based). How does your average working adult or school age child employ these recommendations while navigating through the multiple food choices presented to them on a daily basis? I still can't do this myself! Using analogies like "size of a deck of cards" for meat servings and "size of a tennis ball" for carbohydrate servings are helpful. But quantifying nutrient consumption to this degree is exhausting for people who do it, and unrealistic for the population at large.

For these reasons, I have employed two specific techniques when constructing the 6-Step Diet to ensure practicality and feasibility for the average person on the diet. I refer to these as *food availability* and *brand selection*. *Food availability* refers to making dietary recommendations based upon what your average person in a given society (Western society in our case) may have access to in his daily. For example, we don't generally eat pyramids, so you won't see that on the 6-Step Diet. *Brand Specification* refers to differentiating between specific common brand name items which, although may appear similar on the surface, contain very different nutritional properties.

Our goal is to avoid abstractions and focus on the high yield, tangible weight loss recommendations that do not require too much thought. Our lives are complicated enough as is, our food selection shouldn't be. Below is a list of common foods and brand name items along with their appropriate category designation. This list has been often referred to as a *grocery store list* by my patients. It will help you make good choices in selecting over-the-counter foods when you go shopping. Each item has been thoroughly scrutinized to meet criteria Category 1 criteria for our diet. Enjoy!

Category 1 Salad Dressing

Maple Grove Farms® Sugar Free Balsalmic Vinaigrette
Maple Grove Farms® Sugar Free Rasberry Vinaigrette
South Beach Diet® Ranch Dressing
Ken's Steakhouse® Light Caesar
Wishbone® Salad Spritzers (all flavors)
Waldon Farms® Calorie Free Dressing (all flavors)
Vinegar and olive oil (any brand)

Category 1 Frozen Meals

South Beach Diet® Garlic & Herb Chicken with Green Beans Almondine
South Beach Diet® Garlic Sesame Beef
South Beach Diet® Caprese Style Chicken with Broccoli & Cauliflower
Lean Cuisine® Steak Tips with Portabella Mushrooms
Lean Cuisine® Roasted Turkey & Vegetables
Lean Cuisine® Roasted Garlic Chicken
Weight Watchers® *Smart Ones*® Salisbury Steak Bistro Selections™
Weight Watchers® *Smart Ones*® Roast Beef Bistro Selections™
Cincinnati's Famous Skyline Chili® Original Recipe

Category 1 Common Beverage Brands

Diet caffeine free soda (*Coke*®, *Pepsi*®, *Sprite*®, *7-Up*®...)
Nestea® Diet Lemon Ice Tea
Snapple® Diet Ice Tea (any flavor)
Crystal Light® Ice Tea (any flavor)
Arizona® Diet Ice Tea (any flavor)
Tropicana® Sugar Free Lemonade, Orangeaid, and Fruit Punch
Minute Maid® Light Lemonade
Fresca® Sparkling Flavored Soda (any flavor)
Vault® Zero Citrus Sugar Free Hybrid Energy Soda
Club soda (any brand)
Tonic water (any brand)
Propel® Fitness Water (any flavor)
Fruit2O® No Calories (any flavor)
Clear Excellence® Sparkling Flavored Beverage (any flavor)
6-StepWeight Loss™ fiber mixed fruit drink

Category 1 Common Sauce & Salsa Brands

Heinz® Carb One Ketchup
Yellow mustard (any brand)
Dijon mustard (any brand)
Spicy brown mustard (any brand)
Worcesterchire sauce (any brand)
A-1® Low Carb Steak Sauce
Tobasco® Pepper Sauce original flavor
Hunts® No Sugar Added Spaghetti Sauce
Carb Options® Garden Style Spaghetti Sauce
Bella Faniglia® (BF) Marinara Sauce
Bella Faniglia® (BF) Arrabiata Sauce
Le Roselli's® Marinara Spaghetti Sauce
Le Roselli's® Marinara Pizza Sauce
Taco Bell® Thick & Chunky Salsa
Newman's Own® All Natural Chunky Salsa
Pace® Chunky Salsa
Pace® Picante Sauce
Santa Fe® Black Bean Dip

Category 2 Breads and Wraps

(one slice/wrap is equal to one Category 2 serving)

Nature's Own® Double Fiber
Nature's Own® White Wheat
Banditero® Lo Carb Tortilla
La Tortilla Factory® Lo Carb Tortilla
Mission® Lo Carb Tortilla

Visit www.6stepweightloss.com for latest updates to list of approved foods.

Taste Appeal: Eating foods that taste like cardboard is certainly one way of losing weight. However, we would prefer that weight loss be a more enjoyable and sustainable experience. We have gone the extra step to ensure that the foods on the 6-Step Diet are diverse and highly palatable.

Finding foods that have the right balance of optimal nutrition and taste appeal is challenging. Bad tasting healthy food (raw spinach) leads to poor compliance. Good tasting unhealthy food (burger 'n fries) leads to poor weight loss. In addition to the scrutiny mentioned earlier, taste testing is an important component of our *multi-dimensional nutritional analysis technique.* All the foods recommended on our diet have been taste tested by our staff and our patients.

Patients are also surveyed on a continual basis to see what new foods they would like to see on the diet. Based on these results, we attempt to find compatible products in the grocery store. If unavailable, then we may develop those products ourselves at our center. For example, a common request among our patients initially was more availability of breakfast foods. We did not find very much in the grocery store, so we made available our own brand of oatmeal, breakfast cereal, and pancake mix that met both our nutritional and taste requirements.

Step 4: Cognitive Principles

Remember how I told you unhealthy weight is a multi-factorial disease. In this chapter, you're going to learn about how specific cognitive barriers may have prevented you from losing weight in the past. We have thus far reviewed the importance of having a good medical exam and screening done by your doctor. This will ensure there are no medical barriers standing in the way of your weight loss and will also give you medical clearance to pursue active weight management. We have also gone over some important scientific concepts and physiology involved in weight management as well as reviewed the 6-Step Diet.

A cognitive barrier can be defined as a mental misperception that acts to twist or misalign your understanding of something. The end result is essentially self-deception and misinterpretation of the facts. Psychologists often use cognitive therapy on their patients with clinical depression or clinical anxiety. Cognitive therapy basically involves retelling the story of a certain event to better represent the facts. We all have a tendency to overly generalize or delete positive aspects of certain bad experiences when we want to feel bad about ourselves for something.

An example might be a college student who performs poorly on an exam and later tells himself, "I'm stupid, I'll never do well in school." By saying this to himself a number of times he sets up a cognitive barrier for himself to prevent academic success. Subconsciously, he has set up this new thinking to represent a false perception of reality. This is absolutely a wrong way to think, and if he does not crawl over the mental barrier he's created for himself his perceived reality may even come true! This is known as a "self-fulfilled prophesy."

The correct way to think about his recent poor test score would be the following:

a) I'm obviously smart enough to be in college so I'm not stupid.

b) Everyone fails a test now and then, even the best students.

c) What did I do wrong that I can correct in the future to prevent this from happening again?

The above statements represent the same story of the student's poor test performance but are actually much more accurate in representing the facts of what happened. By focusing on reality, this story eliminates emotional biases and prevents a cognitive barrier from forming.

The most important cognitive barrier you may have regarding weight loss is the thinking that, "I've failed so many times in the past, I'll never lose weight." This type of thinking is not only inaccurate but very destructive. You are responding emotionally to prior failure and are distorting reality. You have to stop thinking this way before you can move on with your weight loss. This is very important!

The reason you failed before is because you went about it the wrong way, not because you can't do it. This book will provide you with the correct methodology and this time you will succeed with both weight loss and weight loss maintenance. Remember, unhealthy weight is multifactorial, and you probably approached it only with diet and/or exercise alone in the past. Now you know that there are other steps involved.

Most patients who come to me for help with their weight have tried various diets in the past and have failed numerous times with either weight loss or maintenance of weight lost. They usually are discouraged and come to me as a last ditch effort to accomplish what they perceive as "the impossible." So you can imagine that I spend a fair amount of time correcting their thinking with cognitive therapy.

I had a patient come to me with a BMI of 40 (severe obesity) who told me that she was doing everything right but not losing the weight. She was on a calorie counting diet and stated that she was only taking in 1200 calories/day and walking about 2 miles/day five days a week. I enrolled her in my program and did a thorough medical screening which showed there was nothing wrong with her body or metabolism that was preventing weight loss. So, I confronted her about this and discovered that the problem was not with her body, but with her mind. "There was no spoon *(The Matrix)*."

I explained to her that it was impossible for her not to lose weight if she was indeed only taking in 1200 calories and on top of that exercising regularly. I reviewed with her Einstein's Theory of The Law of Conservation of Energy which tells us that energy cannot be created or destroyed. It only changes from one form to another. Calories act as little energy molecules in our body, and if we consume more than we use our body converts the extra calories into the form of fat cells for storage. So, either she was wrong in what she was telling me, or Einstein was wrong! When hearing the story told to her in this way she broke down in tears and then began admitting to me the things she had done wrong in the past. She also admitted that she was convinced it was impossible for her to ever lose weight. She actually believed this, as if something in the heavens predetermined she would always be heavy and there was nothing she could do about it! Currently, she has graduated from our program and left still about 50 pounds lighter. Her success underscores the importance of recognizing and eliminating cognitive barriers for a weight loss program to succeed.

Now that you know that weight loss is certainly in your grasp, particularly if you are using this book, let's talk about another disturbing, but common cognitive barrier. This one deals specifically with misperceptions of overweight as part of one's self-definition instead of as a medical condition that can be treated.

We generally use various characteristics to help our minds define and classify ourselves as well at other people. You may classify a person as tall or short; blond hair or dark hair; blue eyes or brown eyes; and fat or thin. It is this last classification as "fat or thin" where the problem lies. Your weight is in every respect a modifiable aspect of yourself and your being. All of the other classifications in the previous list are genetically determined, not permanently modifiable, and not considered disease states.

When you start looking at unhealthy weight for what it is, a disease, and not simply as a personal characteristic trait of your body, you open the door for change and improvement. You will realize that you need to play an active role in your own weight management. This is the case for most diseases out there.

For example, a diabetic patient is expected to play an active role in the management of his disease. This role often includes: taking medication, measuring blood sugars regularly, dietary modification, getting routine blood tests done, etc. The diabetic wouldn't accept his diabetes as just part of his body, like he would his height or his hair color for example, and do nothing about it (at least I hope he wouldn't)!

Unhealthy weight is a disease, and it has reached epidemic proportions in our country. Unhealthy weight results in about 300,000 deaths per year in this country alone and the rate continue to rise. Take a look around you next time you are at the grocery store or shopping mall. Count the first twenty adults you see and calculate how many of those appear overweight or obese to you. I bet you'll get at least 50% almost every time.

The bottom line of this chapter is this. Unhealthy weight IS a disease and CAN be treated. This is the new story to replace whatever story you had convinced yourself of in the past regarding your weight. We need to actively accept that unhealthy weight is a disease on both the individual and societal level and that this disease can be treated like many other common diseases out there. This book is your first step toward that end. Now that we got this all straightened out, let's move on!

Step 5:
Behavioral Principles

In this chapter we're going to deal with another very important element of the 6-Step Weight Loss Program known as behavioral modification. Behavioral modification is crucial to weight loss success but it is often overlooked by your routine dieter (30,31). Your behavior is basically defined as your way of acting or reacting in your environment. Believe it or not, there are many environmental cues constantly acting around you causing you to behave in a repeated, conditioned way that may be sabotaging your weight loss success. For the sake of brevity, I'm going to focus on the aspects of behavioral modification which I feel are the most practical and which have thus far worked out well for my patients. We're going to break this topic up into three subgroups:

1) Eating cues

2) Activity modification

3) Social support

Eating Cues

Conditional reflexes play an important role in determining our behavior. Our bodies and minds are constantly responding to various environmental cues that influence us in different ways. The 19th century Russian scientist Ivan Pavlov was the first to demonstrate the presence of environmental conditioning in his experiment on dogs.

Pavlov did an experiment involving dogs where he rang a bell every time he fed the dogs. After a while, the sound of the bell became the environmental cue for the dogs to eat, and they would salivate readying themselves for a meal every time they heard its sound. The bell cued them to eat even when food was not present.

Let's consider some examples of how our own environment affects us in particular ways. Certain color schemes may change your mood and make you feel a certain way. Soft, brightly mixed colors tend to be uplifting; whereas, dark, ashy colors can be depressing. Slow, rhythmic background music played in grocery stores cues you to slow down your pace. This may mean you spend more money in the store. In the case of ex-smokers, meeting old smoking buddies or visiting old smoking hangouts deliver many cues to have a smoke. This leads to an overwhelming temptation to smoke again. There exist many different environmental triggers that stimulate you to want to eat, even at times when you are not hungry.

These cues can be obvious things like feeling hungry after watching the cooking channel or having a "Big Mac® Attack" after seeing a McDonalds® commercial. You don't need my help identifying and dealing with these type of cues. I would like to focus on helping you find your own personal Pavlovian Bell, so to speak. That is to say, Pavlov was able to associate something completely unrelated to food like a bell tone to appetite stimulation. Each one of us has at least one or two crucial cues that act on us daily and cause us to desire food even when we're not hungry. These cues often have nothing to do with food itself and thus act as our own personal Pavlovian Bell driving us to eat. Once you discover your own Pavlovian Bell and modify your response to it accordingly you'll be amazed as to how much easier weight loss and weight loss maintenance will be. This is an important component of The 6-Step Plan and should be taken seriously. Remember, unhealthy weight is multi-factorial, and we're going to attack it at every angle and therefore conquer it in the end!

In my experience with patients trying to lose weight, the most common Pavlovian Bells are the internal emotions of fatigue, boredom, depression, and stress. These emotional states are very powerful forces and can make or break your weight loss effort. All of us experience at least one of the above emotional states on a consistent basis in our daily lives. They cause us to want to eat. I think the reason is because high caloric, quick-fix food gives us an immediate escape from the above negative emotions. Over time our eating behavior has been adapted to accepting these states as eating cues, thus forming our own personal Pavlovian Bell.

My personal Pavlovian Bell is stress. I have two kids, a thriving medical practice, and an adventurous wife. I'm rarely bored. Fatigue and depression are also unusual for me. However, stress (both the good kind and the bad) is quite common and is a powerful force affecting my eating behavior. My first instinct when feeling stressed is to grab a quick-fix snack, which usually ends up being about 600 calories when I'm done. The way I've dealt with this is by keeping low calorie snacks around me during anticipated stressful situations, like long car trips with the kids. I now grab **a** diet soda and a *6-Step* Fudge Graham Bar when I am stressed and end up consuming 150 calories instead of 600.

There are a number of common external eating cues as well. These include sitting down in a movie theater, watching the big game on tv, or staying in on a rainy day. I think we're all familiar with the different type of cravings these situations bring about. Personally, my biggest external Pavlovian Bell is going to the movies. I immediately crave a big tub of popcorn with massive amounts of that liquid heaven you pour over it at the butter counter! It doesn't matter if I'm going to the movies right after dinner or on an empty stomach. It's always the same. Can you guess what I do to get around this situation? Let's just say my wife usually brings her big purse with her when we go to the movies.

What's your personal Pavlovian Bell? Try taking a few days and focus on the different environmental or emotional cues that bring you to eat even when you're not hungry. When you discover this about yourself you will have taken a big step toward weight loss. You can modify your response to these various cues to significantly reduce your calorie intake thereby taking control of your eating behavior. Maybe you'll snack on diet soda and a Fudge Graham Bar like me. Maybe you'll chew gum instead or keep a tape player around and listen to your favorite song to make you forget about food. If you crave chips and a burger when you watch the game, try buying an assortment of raw veggies and keeping it out before the game begins. You'll naturally reach for it if it's right in front of you. As time goes on, you will have turned your modified response into a habit, and it will get easier and easier to avoid the unnecessary calorie intake when your Pavlovian bell rings.

Activity Modification

Now, let's talk a little bit about activity modification, the second important behavioral principle in weight loss. As Americans, we live in one of the most modern, technologically advanced countries in the world. However, it's no coincidence that Americans are also among the most overweight people in the world. We live in a society of elevators, automobiles, remote controls, automatic doors, etc. These as well as other conveniences of the modern world can trap your weight loss effort by offering too much comfort and encouraging laziness (32). Physical activity (and hence healthy calorie burn) has essentially been engineered out of our society. Consider the following examples.

How many of us have spent an extra five minutes in the car looking for the closest parking space at the grocery store or mall? By doing so we are wasting time, gas, and money (gas is very expensive these days) as well as missing out on a very easy opportunity to burn calories (33). In most buildings elevators are so fast and comfortable that most people reflexively look to use them instead of the stairs.

My wife and I were in an airport one day going from the gate to the customs area which was about 300 meters away. We chose to walk instead of using the moving platform. Needless to say, we were one of the first people to arrive in customs having passed the 90% of people who chose the moving platform (most of whom were standing instead of walking). By over-relying on modern technology to do many of our day to day activities, we miss out on many opportunities to be more physically active and burn more calories. Simple lifestyle modifications in our daily lives go a long way in helping us lose weight and helping us keep it off (34).

One quick note on modern technology though, advancements are made that can actually enhance not hinder our weight loss. One such example is the use of *BodyTogs®*. *BodyTogs®* are anatomically designed resistance sleeves worn under daily wear clothing that enhance calorie burn with practically every movement. Every time you go shopping, walk the dog, run errands, go to work, etc. you end up burning an extra calorie here and extra calorie there so that by the end of the day it's equal to a mile run. Using *BodyTogs®* is a great way to use technology to actually improve weight loss. It will enhance your daily calorie burn by actually giving you a calorie burning workout, without needing to set aside extra time in the day to "workout." More information on *Body-Togs®* can be found at www.bodytogs.com.

Trying to maximize physical effort in your daily life is a practical and easy way to help boost your body's metabolism. Your body will burn calories during times you are used to being inactive. Think of this as the extra credit of weight loss. Remember, unhealthy weight is multifactorial, and we need to hit it at every angle to have long term success. Let those people who really need the modern conveniences be the ones to use them. People with small children or who are medically injured should be the ones using elevators and parking close to buildings.

If you make it a habit to park further away, you'll not only do more walking in a day, but you'll probably get fewer dents in your car too. If you're ever at a grocery store and all the close spots are empty, you'll know that the other people in the store have read this book, and maybe you can strike up a conversation with them. You should also always use stairs whenever you are able. Believe me, it's a great way to burn calories. One of my successful weight loss patients takes 15 minutes during his lunch break every day and walks up and down the stairs in his building. These are easy modifications you can make in your daily activity that will go a long way for you in the long run, particularly with weight loss maintenance.

So, you now know to always park your car far away from your destination and to always use the stairs. What other activity modifications could you make in your day to day life to get more extra credit? Everyone has a different daily routine; think of an activity you can implement on your own. It will be time well spent. Maybe you can spend time pacing while on the phone, do more of the housework yourself instead of using a cleaner, mow your own lawn, etc. As for me, I wrote 60% of this book standing using the kitchen counter instead of sitting at the table!

Regular exercise is also an important part of weight management and good health in general. The American Heart Association recommends exercising at least four days a week for at least 30 minutes a day. This will not only help boost your metabolism but also improve your overall cardiovascular fitness, which basically means your heart will pump more efficiently even when not exercising. Even in people with normal weight, an inactive lifestyle is an independent risk factor for heart disease. So you can tell your skinny friends that regular exercise will add years to their lives too. I recommend a good aerobic activity for my patients at three to four times a week, an activity that gets their heart rate up and makes them sweat. That might be accomplished through a brisk walk, a jog, 30 minutes on the exercise bike, a game of tennis, a swim, etc. Adding some resistance training (push-ups, sit-ups, arm curls, etc.) to your regimen for about 10 minutes twice a week will also be beneficial. Resistance training will add lean muscle mass to your body and help you burn more calories at rest since lean muscle requires more calories for daily maintenance than fat.

There are no more special details you need to know about exercise. You don't need to buy any fancy machines or weight loss gadgets, unless you want to. See what sport or exercise regimen fits best in your daily life and just implement that about four days a week. You can also use *BodyTogs*® during your exercise regimen for added calorie burn. Some of my patients take their dog out for an extra 15 minutes during their walk to meet their exercise quota. Others have tennis buddies they meet on a regular basis. Lots of options, pick something that's realistic for you and stick to it.

Social Support

Let's talk about the final topic under behavior modification: developing a social support system. Don't even think about trying to lose weight in secret! Many people hide the fact that they are dieting because of embarrassment about their weight. If you do this, it may certainly impair your chance for long term success. It is important that those around you are aware of your weight loss effort so they can support you along the way. You'll be surprised at how much your family and close friends will support you once they know you are on a structured weight loss plan.

There will be times where you experience temptation and perhaps you might occasionally cheat on your diet. That is completely natural for anyone! However, you will need an external support system of people around to give you encouragement and moral support during those difficult times. Reassurance from those around you will equip you to deal with temptation when it comes along. It will also help minimize your losses during times you gave in and cheated. This will make it easier to get back on the wagon. We are only human, and small failures here and there are part of our existence. It is how you recover from those tough times that will influence your weight loss success in the end.

Now, you may come across that occasional pushy relative or colleague who is always encouraging you to eat and to give up all that weight loss stuff! Just tell them that you are following your doctor's orders (coming straight from myself, Dr. Virji), and that you don't want to end up as just another statistic. Let them know that unhealthy weight kills 300,000 people a year in this country and you are determined not to be one of those people. Unhealthy weight increases your risk for developing heart disease, stroke, cancer, stomach ulcers, and chronic infections, to name a few. Remember, you are the one (not that pushy relative or colleague of yours) who will face the consequences of letting your weight get out of control. So remember to just brush away those comments if you come across them and move on! Overall, you will find these types of people to be in the minority. Almost everyone else will support you.

You now know the major behavioral techniques which you need to lose weight and to keep it off. You need to find your eating cues and deal with them appropriately; modify your daily activities to work for you not against you; and develop a social support system for reinforcement. Pretty easy, right! Many studies out there show the positive effect of behavioral modification in long term weight loss; so take this part of your program seriously. Go ahead and start making these adjustments in your daily life; the only thing you have to lose is weight! Let's move on.

Step 6:
Weight Loss Maintenance

Congratulations! You've made it this far. You now know all you need to know to lose weight successfully. No fancy gadgets, fad diets, or hocus pocus necessary.

Step one: any medical barriers will be wiped away with your complete physical exam (CPE) and physician consultation. **Step two:** you understand the important neurologic hormones involved in controlling your weight and how to take control of them. You also know how to calculate your BMI and ideal body weight. **Step three:** You know the ins and outs of the clinically proven 6-Step Weight Loss Diet and how it helps you enhance your fat burning hormones and reduce your fat storing hormones. **Step four:** You've broken down cognitive barriers that have sabotaged your weight loss in the past. **Step five:** you've modified your behavior to work for you not against you to achieve weight loss. Now it's time for step six, the most important of them all: weight loss maintenance. We're going to divide this step into four categories as follows:

Goal setting

6-Step Weight Loss Maintenance Diet

Weight surveillance

Medical surveillance

Goal Setting

Rome wasn't built in a day! You will not achieve your ideal body weight overnight. Your weight loss will be gradual. Anyone who tells you otherwise is trying to sell you something. The good news is that if you stick to the principles in this book your weight loss will be permanent! Setting appropriate attainable goals is the first step to successful weight loss maintenance.

Let's go back to chapter two for a moment. Your body has this mechanism by which it tries to pull you back to a certain pre-set weight once you begin weight loss. It tries to accomplish this by means of a powerful neuro-hormone called leptin. Once your fat cells shrink and begin producing less leptin for your brain, your hypothalamus gets very irritated and works hard at stimulating your appetite trying to get you to return to the previous weight. You have to accept this as part of your body's natural physiology to preserve itself, and you have to work around it.

Studies have shown that with as little as a 10% loss of body weight you can achieve significant health benefits in multiple areas. This is a great starting point and will help us deal with leptin! Your weight management plan needs to be divided into two cycles: weight loss and weight loss maintenance. These are two very distinct things.

You will start with a weight loss cycle which begins after you put this book down. For your weight loss cycle you will work toward losing 10% of your body weight in about a three month period. For most people this will be between one and three pounds a week. You will successfully apply what you learned in steps one through five to achieve this goal. You will be losing your weight from every possible angle which will be a change from what you've done in the past, and you'll find that meeting this goal is easier than you think. It is important to follow each of the individual steps to the letter without cheating. Your initial goal weight will unlikely be your dream weight or ideal body weight. Remember, it's a marathon and this is just the first few miles.

After losing 10% of your body weight, your leptin receptors will be charged and ready to try and sabotage your weight loss effort. If you continue to run a full-court-press against your weight now, your leptin receptors will catch you in a crossfire leading back to the road of unhealthy weight(figure 6). At this point, it's a good idea to slow things down and shift to your first weight loss maintenance cycle. Your weight loss maintenance cycle will also last about one to two months.

It is very important to understand the difference between weight loss and weight loss maintenance. During weight loss maintenance your primary focus is on NOT regaining weight. This is very different than losing weight. By focusing on not regaining weight you are giving your body time to readjust to its new internal hormonal environment. At the same time, you are readying yourself for the battle with leptin which happens to be at its height during the first 10% weight loss mark. You must realize that your goal is different in the weight loss maintenance cycle than in the weight loss cycle, and you must exercise patience if you want to achieve long term success.

Weight loss maintenance is less gratifying and socially rewarding than weight loss which is why it is so often neglected. During weight loss your clothes become loose, friends are noticing the difference and making comments about you, and you generally feel great about yourself. These benefits are generally absent during weight loss maintenance leading you to forget about its importance. Do not fall into this trap! This is the time to stand your ground until reinforcements arrive. Focus on keeping your weight where it is for about one to two months and avoid any guilt that you've stopped moving forward for a while. This is all part of the plan. During this time, your hypothalamus will eventually get the idea that this new weight is here to stay. It will downgrade its number of leptin receptors to accept this new lower concentration of leptin as its baseline and stop pushing you so hard to regain the weight (figure 7).* Once this is achieved, after about one to two months, you will be able to re-enter another weight loss cycle if desired.

Remember, all you need is a 10% loss of body weight to get a significant health benefit and add years to your life. When you've reached this point you have already achieved success! However, if you wish to pursue further weight loss, then by all means, let's keep going and enter weight loss cycle number two. Just remember, you need every step in this book to make your changes permanent. Skipping steps will only harm you in the end. To enter weight loss cycle number two you'll need to start with step one again and take a trip to your doctor for another medical screening. Since we've already gone through one cycle we'll refer to this as *medical surveillance*, covered later in this chapter.

* The theory of hypothalamic receptor modulation over a period of time is generally the author's inference. The science of leptin physiology is relatively new and many studies continue in this area. It is well-accepted in the scientific community that slow-steady weight loss is safer and more sustainable than quick, immediate weight loss. In addition, receptor modulation in various organ systems secondary to various stimuli is a common physiologic phenomenon in the body. These are the basis of the author's inference regarding long-term hypothalamic receptor modulation.

6-Step Weight Loss Maintenance Diet

All right, let's discuss how your diet is going to change during your weight loss maintenance cycle. This part of the program is actually quite simple. Let's begin with a brief review of the 6-Step Weight Loss Diet.

The 6-Step Weight Loss Diet has been designed to enhance your fat burning hormones and reduce your fat storing hormones. By selecting the *right* foods and food combinations you do have control of these hormones. For this reason, you can enjoy a large variety of foods while on the diet and still lose weight. Other aspects of the diet including considerations of food availability, brand specification, and taste appeal make it that much easier and convenient to follow. Remember this is the "80% knowledge and 20% effort weight loss diet and lifestyle." You have effectively replaced a large part of the effort with your newly acquired knowledge and your use of our *multi-dimensional nutritional analysis technique* to guide your food selection. If you follow the diet and count your categories correctly, you will likely find that this is one of the easiest diets you have ever tried!

As human beings we naturally crave a variety of foods and diets that tend to limit choice for long periods of time tend to fail for most people. During this part of the diet I would like to bring in some of those foods you may have missed during your weight loss phase, namely those notorious *Category 3* foods. During weight loss maintenance you essentially continue the 6-Step Weight Loss Diet as you have been, but you are now allowed up to two servings of *Category 3* foods per day. Maybe you are missing those French fries or popcorn….pizza or pasta….rice or potato chips. No problem! Bring in up to two servings of these foods a day. One day you may enjoy a slice of pizza and a bowl of rice. Another day you may enjoy some spaghetti and a slice of garlic bread. Just be sure to continue the rest of the parts of the diet exactly as you have been before. Continue to enjoy two *Category 2's* and two *Category 4's* each day with unlimited *Category 1's*.

By continuing to eat along the general template of the 6-Step Weight Loss Diet your body will continue to benefit from higher levels of fat burning hormones and lower levels of fat storing hormones. Remember that the diet is physiologic and works with your body, not against it to lose weight. At the same time, the added *Category 3* options in moderation (limited to two servings a day) will appease your taste buds and give you the variety you need to help you keep your new weight loss diet and lifestyle permanent.

During this part of the program you should see your weight stabilize without any major fluctuations up or down. You will, however, need to monitor your weight closely. Let's talk about how to do that.

Weight Surveillance

In order to maintain your weight successfully you need to accurately track your weight. Weighing yourself at various times during the day can sometimes be misleading. Weight may fluctuate throughout the day depending on such things as clothing, food intake, and time of the month for women.

A better way to go about weight surveillance is by weighing

yourself everyday *at the same time*. I recommend that once you have entered weight loss maintenance that you weigh yourself every day, in the morning, in your pajamas, after you have gone to the bathroom. This is a better, more accurate way to track your weight and also helps to avoid the common pitfall of "scale obsession." Many people weigh themselves multiple times a day, and the number that pops up on the scale basically determines their mood for the rest of the day. This number is not only misleading but will lead you to a lot of anxiety since it will naturally fluctuate from hour to hour and day to day. You need to break out of this habit! Think of it this way, drinking a 16oz bottle of water will cause that number to go up one pound. That extra weight is obviously not coming from your fat cells. When you relieve yourself thirty minutes later that weight will conveniently disappear.

Go out and buy a good scale. Weigh yourself daily exactly as I have recommended, in the morning, in your pajamas, after you have gone to the bathroom. Keep track of that number on a daily basis and watch out for fluctuations. If you notice yourself starting to creep up on the scale, then immediately restart the 6-Step Weight Loss Diet (see chapter 3) for 48 hours, and that weight will quickly disappear.

For example, if you currently weigh 150 lbs and are in weight loss maintenance mode you will be weighing yourself daily (in the morning, in your pajamas, after you've gone to the bathroom). If you start seeing that number creep up, first to 150.5 lbs, then 150.8 lbs, then 151.3

lbs…then you know to jump right back on the 6-Step Weight Loss Diet for 48 hours. That weight will disappear as quickly as it came on! The reason for this is that those initial two pounds or so do not represent added weight from fat cells. They represent added weight from water and glycogen, which is the storage form of glucose. Glycogen can be burned quickly and easily by restarting the diet, and you'll be back to 150 lbs in no time.

Also keep in mind that not all scales are the same. Weighing yourself at home and at the doctor's office may give you different numbers each time. That is not important. What is important is that your daily weights at home are compatible with your weight management goal.

Medical Surveillance

Let's talk about medical surveillance. To do this we need to go back to step one for a moment. If you had any abnormal tests during your complete physical exam (CPE) including: high blood pressure, high bad cholesterol, low good cholesterol, elevated liver enzymes, or elevated glucose then the first thing you'll need once you've achieved a 10% weight loss is to set up a follow-up appointment with your doctor (if all of these were normal and you have no other chronic medical problems you can skip this part). Ask him or her to retest any of the prior abnormal test results. You will see a significant change for the better! We know that unhealthy weight negatively affects just about every organ system in the body and with your initial weight loss you will see the difference for yourself. No need to take my word for it, seeing is believing! If you are on a medication for blood pressure, diabetes, heartburn, arthritis pain, or high cholesterol there is a possibility you can come off your medication or at least lower the dosage. After all, shedding pounds often helps you to shed medications too. You can only do this with the help of your doctor though and should never try to change your medications on your own.

Experiencing the improvement in any of the weight related medical diseases generally acts as a very strong positive reinforcement tool. I've had to stop a number of medications on my weight loss patients, and they love it! This will help ensure your long term success and weight loss maintenance. By seeing the total benefit for your health overall, not just your self-esteem, it will be easier for you to combat future temptation toward overeating or inactivity. It will also ready you for another weight loss cycle if that is in your long term plan.

Conclusion

Congratulations! You've almost finished the book. You are now fully armed to combat your weight and never have it overtake you again. And you've learned it all in record time. By utilizing the 6-Step Weight Loss program you will be applying the best that both the old science and new science of weight management have to offer. The choice to move on and take action is now yours. Don't hesitate and don't look back!

In the year 2000, this country spent $117 billion dollars in treating obesity and obesity related diseases (35). That's money that could have been spent on tackling the unemployment issue, expanding health care to those without coverage, and feeding needy children. Speaking of children, the crisis of unhealthy weight has not left them untouched. Thirty percent of our nation's children and adolescents have reached the unhealthy weight mark, an all time high! Diseases like high blood pressure, high cholesterol, and diabetes which have traditionally been exclusive to the adult population have now hit our children at alarming levels (36). It was a very disturbing moment for me the first time I had to recommend a diabetic medication for an obese 10 year old.

Always remember that unhealthy weight is a medical condition, not a character trait. It needs to be addressed at every angle in order to be controlled. Each step in this book has a specific purpose, and each step must be understood and utilized thoroughly. If you didn't understand a certain section of the book, then go back and reread that section. There is no shame in that. Like my colleagues in medicine, I had to go through 11 years of training to become a physician. Believe me, during that time I had to reread many sections of many different books before I understood what was being taught.

It has been my privilege to assist you in your weight loss effort. As you can see, treating your weight not only has countless individual benefits, but benefits society as well. Be confident that you now know how to lose weight successfully and keep it off. Leave all excuses and cognitive barriers behind. You simply don't have time for them. Today is your day. Begin with changing your life, then go out and change the world! I wish you success and good health.

Bonus Chapter:
Over-the-Counter Diet Aids

Let's talk a moment about over-the-counter weight loss remedies. I would like to briefly mention this topic since my own patients frequently ask about them and since so many people currently use them. As a rule of thumb, you should utilize extreme caution when considering the use of over-the-counter quick fix diet pills! Most of them have not been tested for safety or efficacy, and in reality there is no way of knowing what you are doing to your body. The 6-Step Essentials Nutritional Supplement contains the essential micronutrients you need to support healthy weight loss and fat burning and has been rigorously tested for purity and potency.

Over-the-counter preparations containing the once popular *Ephedra* (or ephedrine) diet supplement have been officially banned in the United States as of April 12, 2004. Ephedra is a naturally occurring amphetamine- like compound extracted from the *Ephedra* species of plants including the ancient Chinese *Ma huang* and *Sida Cordifolia* to name a few. Unregulated Ephedra supplementation has lead to the death of a number of athletes and results in an inappropriately high risk for stroke, heart attack, and sudden death syndrome.

Some common commercial products contain a mixture of herbal preparations including *Garcinia cambogia*, coca seed extract, and caffeine. Few scientific studies are available to corroborate the hefty weight loss claim of many of these preparations. In addition, their side effects may include elevated blood pressure, heart palpitations, and insomnia. Certain aruveidic herbal preparations have shown some modest weight loss benefit. However, a recent study showed that a number of commonly available over-the-counter aruveidic compounds contained potentially harmful levels of lead, mercury, and arsenic (37)!

There are even a number of natural preparations on the market that claim to help you lose weight by modulating your body's leptin or insinuating that they contain leptin. These preparations tend to be quite expensive as well. You should know that orally ingested leptin does not enter the brain and will therefore have no influence on suppressing your appetite. Studies have failed to show a benefit of oral leptin supplementation on weight loss. Trust me, if it were that easy, I'd be the first one to tell you about it! So save your money. You're going to need it in about three months anyway, for your new wardrobe to replace all those large sizes that don't fit you anymore.

I would like to make a special mention of two over-the-counter compounds which have received a lot of recent attention: *Hoodia gordonii* and green tea extract (EGCG). *Hoodia gardonii* comes from a family of plant which is natively grown in the Kalahari Desert of South Africa. The native tribes of the Kalahari Desert are known to chew on the *Hoodia* plant during long hunting excursions in order to suppress their appetite. Small published clinical studies have actually supported claims of modest appetite suppression with no known side effects. The active component of *Hoodia gardonii* is an extract known as P57. Only *Hoodia* known to contain the active P57 ingredient, that is *Hoodia* cultivated in the Kalahari Desert, is believed to have any effect in appetite suppression. The problem lies in the fact that the vast majority of *Hoodia* on the market does not contain P57. Extracts of *Hoodia* that do not contain P57, in addition to non-*Hoodia* species, are currently sold as *Hoodia gardonii*. Purchasing most brands of over-the-counter *Hoodia* would be considered a gamble at best. The *6-Step Weight Loss™ Appetite Control* supplement is made from authentic *Hoodia gardonii* cultivated from the Kalahari Desert. It is one of only a handful of over-the-counter brands that have been tested for potency, purity, quality, and authenticity. *Hoodia* can be a helpful aid to weight loss by helping control appetite and carbohydrate cravings if needed. Best of all, it has no known side effects and is heart healthy.

The green tea extract epigallocatechin gallate (EGCG) is also worthwhile mentioning. EGCG is a nutrient known as a polyphenol. Polyphenols help give green tea leaves and other plants their natural color. Studies on EGCG suggest that it may enhance the body's basal metabolic rate and hence may be useful in long term weight loss. One randomized placebo controlled study showed it to help moderately obese men lose weight and reduce their waist circumference. The studies on EGCG are still relatively new and more studies need to be done before definitive conclusions can be made on its role in weight loss. One important difference involving green tea in general, when compared to other weight loss compounds, is its seemingly positive effect on overall health, independent of weight loss. A recent study conducted in Japan on over 40,000 people showed green tea consumption to be associated with significant reductions in cardiovascular disease as well as significant reductions in early death due to all causes (for these reasons, EGCG has been included in the *6-Step Essentials* Nutritional Supplement) (38). Various other polyphenols found in fruits and vegetables are also believed to play an important role in cancer prevention.

Recipes

The following are original recipes coming from the wonderful 6-Step Weight Loss staff and their family members. All recipes have been reviewed by Dr. Virji and approved for the labeled categories. *Bon apetite!*

From the West
Authentic Italian Ministrone Soup
Greek Pesto Chicken
Homemade Chicken Soup
Eggless Egg Salad
Pizza Pizza

From the East
Jeddah Mediterranean Salad
Chicken Tikka
6-Step Rotti (Indian Flatbread)
Beef Kebabs
Curried Okra
Bhurjee (South Asian Omelet)

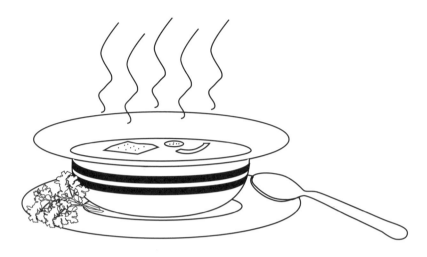

Category 1

Authentic Italian Ministrone Soup

(Dr. Virji favorite)

One head of Romaine lettuce
Two heads of Endivia lettuce
One head of Essccorla lettuce
2 cans kidney beans
3 tbsp olive oil
4 cloves garlic, crushed
3 onions, chopped
6 tomatoes or crushed stewed (blended)
2 cans tomatoes
2 cups water
salt and pepper

Start out by heating oil in a large pot. Add crushed garlic and onions. Saute for 3-4 minutes till onions become transparent. Cut all lettuce heads into big chuncky pieces. Then add the lettuce to the onion mixture. Cook under medium heat until greens wilt down. Add tomatoes and salt & pepper to taste. Bring up to a boil then add kidney beans and water. Bring up to a boil again and allow to simmer for 20-30 minutes.

Serves 4 to 6

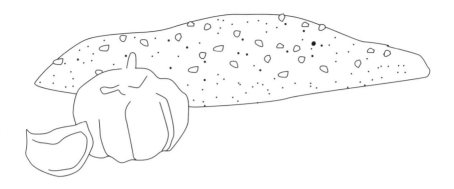

Category 1 and 2

Greek Pesto Chicken

(Dr. Virji favorite)

For the Chicken:
　　1 pound chicken breast cutlets
　　1 cup low fat yogurt
　　ground cumin & corriander (½ tsp each)
　　salt & pepper to taste
　　½ tsp mustard seeds
　　½ tsp sliced ginger
　　2 cloves garlic, sliced

For the Salad:
　　Any variety of pre packaged lettuce
　　cucumber, sliced
　　½ cup pitted kalamata olives, sliced
　　1 tomato, diced
　　salt & pepper to taste
　　1 lemon, juiced

extra virgin olive oil
10 walnuts

For the Pesto:
   1 6 ounce feta cheese, crumbled
   1 bunch italian parsley
   ½ onion,
   1 garlic clove
   10 walnuts
   salt & pepper
   extra virgin olive oil

Marinate the chicken in the above ingredients for up to 30 minutes then grill. Mix salad ingredients together and place onto a serving tray. Blend Pesto ingredients in a blender until a smooth consistency. Layer slices of chicken breast on top of salad with dallops of pesto sauce over chicken. Top off with extra feta cheese and parsley leaves for garnish

Serves 4 to 6 (each serving equals one category 2)

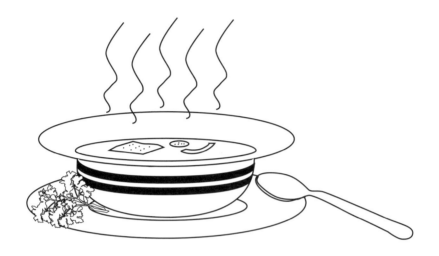

Category 1

Homemade Chicken Soup

1 chicken baked or roasted (or any cooked chicken) cubed
2 cans of chicken broth (or homemade chicken broth)
1 medium yellow onion diced
3 stalks of celery diced
1 or 2 packages frozen broccoli and cauliflower
2 tablespoons dried parsley
Salt & pepper

Bake or roast chicken until almost completely cooked then cube. In a large pot bring the chicken stock up to a boil, add the diced onion and celery and cook for 5 minutes. Shred the cubed chicken and add it to the stock. Add the dried parsley and salt & pepper (to taste). Add the frozen broccoli and cauliflower and cook another 10 minutes.

Serves 6 to 8

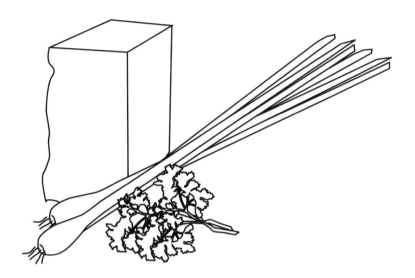

Category 1

Eggless Egg Salad

2 pounds soft tofu
½ cup low fat mayonnaise
3 tbsp Dijon mustard
1 tsp cayenne pepper
½ tsp tumeric powder
1 tbsp chopped flat-leaf parsley
1 tbsp chopped fresh dill
½ cup diced green onions
salt and pepper to taste

Mash tofu with a wooden spoon and put into a mixing bowl. Mix in all of the above ingredients with the mashed soft tofu and stir well. Cover and chill slightly. Serve on a bed of mixed greens topped off with bean sprouts.

Serves 4 to 6

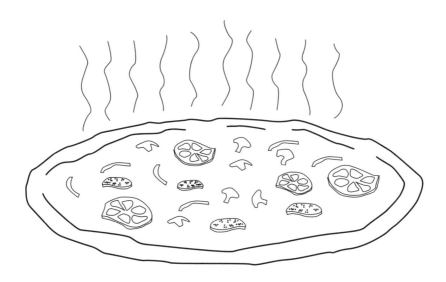

Category 1

Pizza Pizza

1 head cauliflower
1 cup grated low fat mozzarella cheese
2 eggs beaten
½ cup low fat or fat free Italian grated cheese
2 tablespoons parsley flakes
½ teaspoon basil flakes
Le Roselli's® Marinara Pizza Sauce
Salt & Pepper
5 to 6 tablespoons soy flour (optional)
Non stick spray

*Steam the cauliflower until tender in salted water (about 15
minutes). Drain thoroughly. Put the cooked cauliflower in a
food processor or blender and process until smooth (or use a*

potato masher). You should end up with around 3 cups of processed cauliflower. Add the grated mozzarella, Italian grated cheese, beaten eggs to the cauliflower and mix well. Add the parsley flakes and basil, salt and pepper to taste and soy flour.

Spray a cookie sheet or round pizza pan (these can be found in the grocery store – if using round disposable pizza pans you should get two pizzas). Spread the cauliflower mixture as thinly and as evenly as possible. Bake for 7 to 10 minutes at 425 degrees in the middle of the oven (this will allow the cauliflower to settle). Dress the pizza with pizza sauce and your favorite toppings and bake for 10 to 15 minutes or until the cheese melts on top.

Serve this pizza with a big salad with tomatoes, cucumbers, olives and chick peas. Dress the salad with olive oil, salt & pepper and a little lemon juice.

Serves 4 to 6

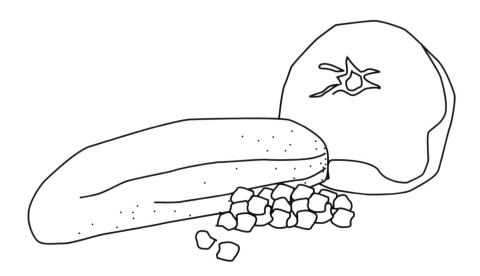

Category 1

Jeddah Mediterranean Salad

(Dr. Virji Favorite)

1 can of garbonzo beans
½ head of lettuce
1 cucumber
2 tomatoes
4 coriander leaves
½ teaspoon of salt
1 lemon
¼ tsp red chili powder

Chop lettuce, tomatoes, cucumber and coriander and mix them together in a salad bowl. Drain out liquid from can of garbonzo beans and add into a pot with 1 cup of water. Add salt

*and chili powder to the pot, mix, and boil for about 10 minutes.
Drain garbonzo beans and add to salad bowl with the beans
on the top. Squeeze over the top one whole lemon and serves.*

Serves 3 to 4

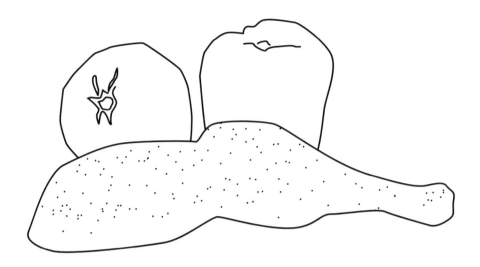

Category 1

Chicken Tikka

2 lbs chicken (legs and quarters)
4 tbs low fat yogurt
1 tbs finely chopped cilantro leaves (about 6 leaves)
3 green chilies
1 tbs tomato puree
1½ tsp salt
2 cloves of garlic (finely chopped)
1 small ginger root (finely chopped)
Olive oil cooking spray
2 medium sized tomatoes
2 bell peppers

Remove skin and excess fat from chicken pieces. Blend green chilies, cilantro leaves, garlic, and ginger into a paste. Then add the paste to a bowel and mix in yogurt, salt, and tomato puree. Add the chicken pieces in and marinate for 1 hour. Then pan fry the chicken over medium heat on lighly coated pan until reddish brown texture is obtained and meat is thoroughly cooked. Remove chicken from pan and add to serving bowel. After all chicken is cooked and moved to serving bowl, add remaining sauce left over from chicken marinade into pan and cook for 2 minutes. Pour over chicken in serving bowl. Garnish with fresh thinly cut tomatoes and bell peppers. Serve with Jeddah Salad (see recipe in this book). You may also serve with 6-Step Rotti (see recipe in this book). Be sure to count each rotti as one Category 2.

Serves 4 to 6

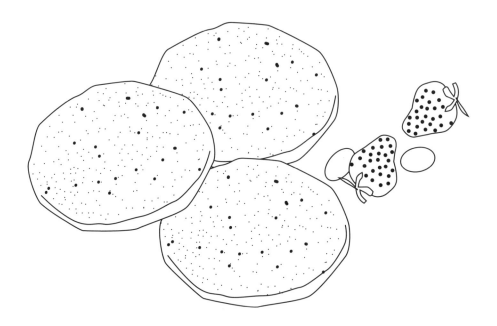

6-Step Rotti (Indian Flatbread)

1 cup soy flour
½ cup buckwheat flour
½ cup vital wheat gluten
cup warm water
tbs olive oil
tbs finely cut cilantro leaves
1 tsp garlic paste
1 tsp salt
olive oil cooking spray

Combine the soy flour, buckwheat flour, wheat gluten, finely cut cilantro leaves, garlic paste, salt, and olive oil into a large mixing bowl. Mix into a pliable dough with warm water adding only 2 tablespoons of water at a time until doughy, non sticky texture is obtained (may lightly coat with whole wheat flour if needed). Knead for 5 minutes then let sit covered with a damp cloth for 30 minutes. Then divide the dough into golf ball size portions. Roll out into flat shaped discs approximately 6 inches in diameter, lightly flouring board as necessary. Cook the discs on a griddle or flat pan (lightly coated with olive oil cooking spray) until the surface appears light brown and bubbly. Turn over and cook other side. You may press the edges of the rotti down with a spatula to help it cook evenly. Repeat with remaining dough and store rottis covered under a damp cloth until finished cooking.

Makes 6-8 rotti's
(each rotti counts as one Category 2)

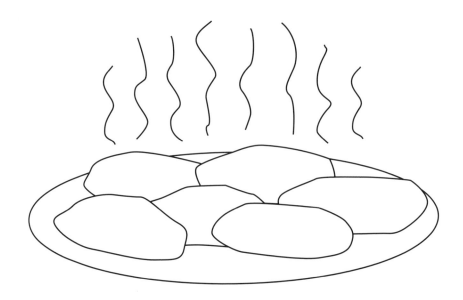

Category 1

Beef Kebabs

2 lbs lean ground beef (90% lean or better)
1 tsp black pepper
1½ tsp ginger powder
1½ tsp red chili powder
½ tsp cardamom powder
½ tsp salt
1 egg, medium size
1 tablespoon olive oil
Olive oil cooking spray

Mix together ground beef, pepper, ginger powder, red chili powder, cardamom powder, salt, and olive oil into a mixing bowl. Break one medium sized egg and add to mixture. Mix ground beef and spices thoroughly by hand for at least two minutes until spices absorbed by meat. Roll kebabs into individual lime shaped patties (have a bowl of warm water ready for hand dipping when rolling kebabs). Grease large frying pan with olive oil cooking spray. Pan fry (avoid deep frying) kebobs over medium heat until browned and thoroughly cooked. Serve with a side of Jeddah Salad (refer to recipe in this book), or side salad if desired.

You may also serve with 6-Step Flat Rotti (refer to recipe in this book), but be sure to count each rotti as one Category 2.

Serves 4 to 6

Curried Okra

16 oz cut okra
1 medium onion, thinly sliced
½ tsp garlic paste
¼ tsp tumeric powder
¼ tsp chili powder
¼ tsp ground cumin
¼ tsp ground corriander
1 tsp salt
1 medium tomato, diced
3 tbsp oil
½ lemon, juiced

Heat oil in pot and sate onions until transparent. Add the okra stirring frequently. Cook under med-high for 5 minutes. Add remaining ingredients except for the lemon. Lower burner to medium. Allow to cook for another 25-30 minutes until okra is soft and no longer sticky. Add freshly squeezed lemon juice and turn off. Allow to sit five minutes before serving. . Serve with a side of Jeddah Salad (refer to recipe in this book) or side salad if desired.

You may also serve with 6-Step Flat Rotti (refer to recipe in this book), but be sure to count each rotti as one Category 2.

Serves 4 to 6

Category 1

Bhurjee (South Asian Omelet)

4 eggs
2 chopped onions
1 chopped tomatos
3 coriander leaves
½ tsp curry powder
¼ tsp tumaric
¼ tsp black pepper
½ tsp garlic paste
¼ tsp salt
1 tbs low fat butter (Smart Balance® Light preferred)

Chop up onions, tomatoes, and coriander leaves and set aside. Whisk together 4 eggs in a bowl and set aside. In a skillet add butter on medium heat. Brown the onions, then add tomatoes, garlic paste, coriander, turmeric, salt, curry powder and black pepper. Sauté for three minutes then add the eggs. Cook until eggs are cooked.

Serves 2 to 3

References

Peeters A, Barendregt JJ, Willekens F, et al, for NEDCOM, the Netherlands Epidemiology and Demography Compression of Morbidity Research Group. Obesity in adulthood and its consequences for life expectancy: a life-table analysis. Ann Intern Med. 2003; 138: 24-32.

Calle, EE, Thun, MJ, Petrelli, JM, et al. Body-mass index and mortality in a prospective cohort of U.S. Adults. N Engl J Med 1999; 341:1097.

National Center for Health Statistics, Centers for Disease Control and Prevention, website www.cdc.gov/nchs/products/pubs/pubd/hestats/obese/obse99.htm (accessed April 20, 2004)

Friedman, XE, Reichmann, SK, Costanzo, PR, et al. Body image partially mediates the relationship between obesity and psychological distress. Obes Res 2002; 10:33-41.

Cohen IA. Nutritional Analysis of popular historical weight-reduction diets. Obes Res 2005; 13:A-139.

Stern L, Nayyar I, Seshadri P, et al. The effects of low-carbohydrate versus conventional weight loss diets in severely obese adults; one-year follow-up of a randomized trial. Ann Int Med 2004; 140:778-785.

Samaha, FF, Iqbal N, Seshadri, P, et al. A low carbohydrate as compared with a low-fat diet in severe obesity. N Engl J Med. 2003;348:2074-2081

Kennedy, A, Gettys, TW, Watson, P, et al. The metabolic significance of leptin in humans: gender-based differences in relationship to adiposity, insulin sensitivity, and energy expenditure. J Clin Endocrinol Metab 1997; 82:1293

Ostlund, RE Jr, Yang, JW, Klein, S, Gingerich, R. Relation between plasma leptin concentration and body fat, gender, diet, age, and metabolic covarities. J Clin Endocrinol Metab 1006; 81:3909.

NHLBI Obesity Education Initiative. Clinical guidelines on the identification, evaluation, and treatment of overweight and obesity in adults: the Evidence Report. NIH Publication No. 98-4083, U.S. Department of Health and Human Services, Public Health Service, National Institutes of Health, National Heart, Lung, and Blood Institute, Bethesda, MD 1998.

Choban, P, Atkinson, R, Moore, BJ. (Shape up America and the American Obesity Association.) Guidance for treatment of adult obesity, 1996: 1996-1998.

US Department of Agriculture, Agriculture Research Service. Data tables: results from USDA's 1994-96 Continuing Survey of Food Intakes by Individuals and 1994-96 Diet and Health Knowledge Survey. ARS Food Surveys Research Group, 1997. http://www.barc.usda.gov/bhnrc/foodsurvey/home.htm (accessed 12 March 2005).

Zemel, Mb, Thompson, W, Milstead, A, et al. Calcium and dairy acceleration of weight loss and fat loss during energy restriction in obese adults. Obes Res. 2004; 12:582-590.

Anderson RS, Chromium: Roles in the regulation of lean body mass and body weight, in *Scientific Evidence for Muskuloskeletal, Bariatric, and Sports Nutrition*, Kohlstadt I, Taylor & Francis, NY, 2006, pp. 174-189.

Wutzke KD and Lorenz H. The effect of L-carnitine on fat oxidation, protein turnover, and body composition in slightly overweight subjects. Metabolism 2004 53(8):1002-6.

Caballero E. Endothelial dysfunction in obesity and insulin resistance: a road to diabetes and heart disease. Obes Res. 2003;11:1278-1289.

Gannon MC, Nuttall JA, Nuttall FQ, et al. Oral arginine does not stimulate an increase in insulin concentration but delays glucose disposal. Am J Clin Nutr 2002;76:1016-22.

Spindel E, Arnold M, Cusack B, et al. Effects of caffeine on anterior pituitary and thyroid function in the rat. J Pharmacol Exp Ther. 1980 Jul;214(1):58-62.

Wutzke KD, Lorenz H. The effect of L-Carnitine on fat oxidation, protein turnover, and body composition in slightly overweight subjects. Metabolism 2004 53(8):1002-6.

Zemel MB, Thompson W, Milstead A, et al. Calcium and dairy acceleration of weight loss and fat loss during energy restriction in obese adults. Obes Res. 2004; 12:582-590.

Kovacs EM, Westerterp-Plantenga MS, Saris WH et al. The effect of the addition of modified guar gum to a low energy semisolid meal on appetite and body weight loss. Int J Obes 2001;25:1.

Arts IC, Hollman PC. Polyphenols and disease risk in epidemiologic studies. Am J Clin Nutr 2005;81(suppl):317S-25S.

Samaha, FF, Iqbal N, Seshadri, P, et al. A low carbohydrate as compared with a low-fat diet in severe obesity. N Engl J Med. 2003;348:2074-2081

Brehm BJ, Seely RJ, Daniels SR. A randomized trial comparing a very low carbohydrate diet and a low calorie-restricted low fat diet on body weight and cardiovascular risk factors in healthy women. J Clin Endocrinol

Lichtman, SW, Pisarska, K, Berman, ER, et al. Discrepancy between self-reported and actual caloric intake and exercise in obese subjects. N Eng J Med 1992; 327:1893

Wing RR, Jeffery RW. Food provision as a strategy to promote weight loss. Obes Res. 2001;9(suppl 4):271S-275S. Abstract

Flechtner-Mors, M, Ditschuneit, HH, Johnson, TD, et al. Metabolic and weight loss effects of long-term dietary intervention in obese patients: four-year results. Obes Res 2000; 8:399.

Wu FB, Willett WC. Optimal diets for prevention of coronary heart disease. JAMA 2002;288:2569-2578.

Rolls BJ. The supersizing of America: Portion size and the obesity epidemic. Nutr Today 2003;38:2:42-49.

Foreyt, JP, Goodrick, GK. Evidence for success of behavior modification in weight loss and control. Ann Intern Med 1993; 119:698. Abstract

Hu, FB, Li, YL, Colditz, GA, et al. Television watching and other sedentary behaviors in relation to risk of obesity and type 2 diabetes melitis in women. JAMA 2003; 289:1785-1791

Levine, JA, Schleusner, SJ, Jensen, MD. Energy Expenditure of nonexercise activity. Am J Clin Nutr 2000; 72:1451.

Anderson, RE, Wadden, TA, Bartlett, SJ, et al. Effects of lifestyle activity vs structured aerobic exercise in obese women. JAMA 1999; 281:335.

Wadden TA, Berkowits RI, Sarwer DB, Prus-Wisniewski R, Steinberg C. Benefits of lifestyle modification in the pharmacologic treatment of obesity: a randomized trial. Arch Intern Med. 2001;161:218-227.

Wolf AM, Colditz GA. Current estimates of the economic cost of obesity in the United States. Obes Res 1998;6:97-106.

Must A, Anderson SE. Effects of obesity on morbidity in children and adolescents. Nutr Clin Care 2003;6:4-12.

Saper RB, Stefanos SN, Paquin J, et al. Heavy metal content of ayurvedic herbal medicine products. JAMA. 2004; 292:2868-2873.

Kuriyama S, Shimazu T, Ohmori K, et al. Green tea consumption and mortality due to cardiovascular disease, cancer, and all causes in Japan. JAMA. 2006;296:1255-1265.

The Skinny Book ~ Second Edition

portant for good heart health and a number of other important physiological functions.

Linolenic Acid: An Omega 3 essential fatty acid. Cannot be made by the body so must be consumed in the diet. Important for good heart health and a number of other important physiological functions.

Low-Fat Diet: A diet strategy involving the strict limitation of dietary fat in order to control energy density and total calorie intake.

Low-Carb Diet: A diet strategy involving the strict limitation of dietary carbohdreate in order to control the body's natural thermogenesis.

Non-Exercise Activity Thermogenesis (NEAT): Calories burned through physical activity not involving volitional exercise. Examples include housecleaning, yardwork, shopping, and occupational activity.

Obesity: A medical condition involving the unhealthy accumulation of fat cells (adipose tissue) in the body. Predisposes an individual to multiple medical conditions including heart disease, diabetes, and cancer. Generally defined as a body mass index ≥ 30. Also may be defined as a waste circumference ≥ 40 in men and ≥ 35 in women.

Thermogenesis: A physiologic process in the body involving the burning of calories to generate heat. An important aspect of weight loss.

Glossary of Terms

Body Mass Index (BMI): A measure of an individual's weight status. Calculated as weight in kilograms divided by height in meters squared.

Cortisol: A hormone secreted by the body's agrenal gland which is involved in glucose regulation and fat deposition

Energy Density: The calorie content of food unit serving. Influenced by the ratio of fat, carbohydrate, protein, and water content of the food.

Glucagon: A hormone secreted by the body's pancreas responsible for breaking down glycogen into glucose for energy utilization.

Growth Hormone: A hormone secreted by the pituaitary gland in the brain which controls muscle growth and metabolism in the adult. Important for holding on to lean muscle during weight loss.

HDL Cholesterol: High density lipoprotein. Good cholesterol.

Insulin: A hormone secreted by the pancreas involved in glucose metabolism and fat synthesis. Generally levels too high in overweight and obese individuals.

LDL Cholesterol: Low density lipoprotein. Bad cholesterol.

Leptin: A hormone secreted by fat cells involved in appetite regulation and metabolism

Linoleic Acid: An Omega 6 essential fatty acid. Cannot be made by the body so must be consumed in the diet. Im-